T'ai Chi for Beginners

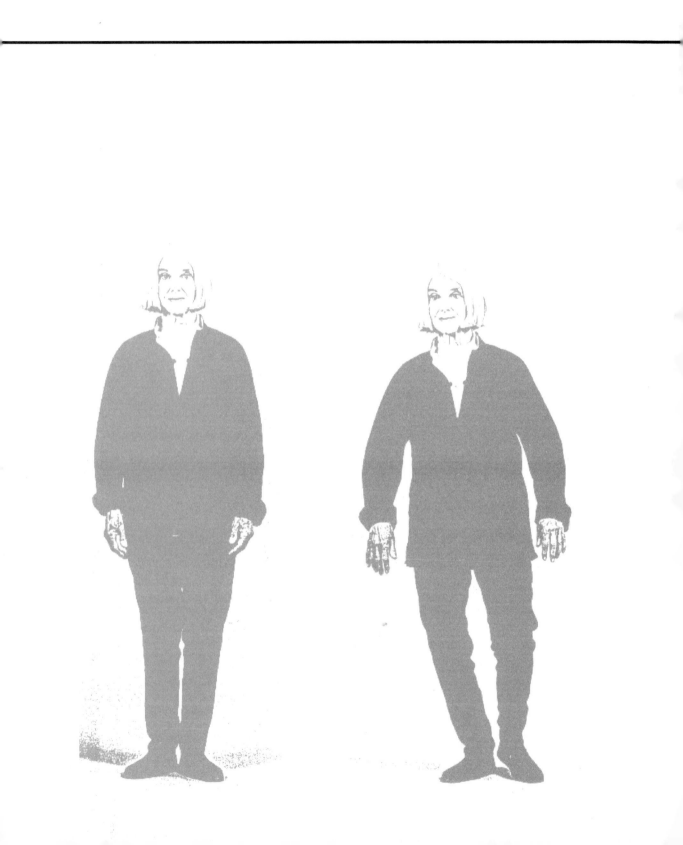

T'AI CHI FOR BEGINNERS

10 MINUTES
TO
HEALTH AND
FITNESS

CLAIRE
HOOTON

PHOTOGRAPHS BY
JAMES STILES

A PERIGEE BOOK

Book design by H. Roberts
Cover design by James R. Harris
Cover photograph by Ed Taylor
Interior photographs by James Stiles

ISBN: 0-399-52207-7

Printed in the United States of America

For my son, Hart

CONTENTS

ACKNOWLEDGMENTS

Many people have helped this book become a reality. Special thanks go to David Myers, who has given me his writer's wisdom and invaluable support, and to my editor, Sheila Curry. I am grateful also to my agent, Nancy Love, who said one day, "Claire, why don't you write a book about T'ai Chi?" Enormous thanks also to the following gifted people for their major contributions: Coco Myers, David Monet, and James Stiles. And to Sarah Wolins, my student and friend, for proofing the positions with me.

And there are those people who did extra uncalled-for favors to assist this venture. Thank you to Cal Pozo, Chris Kraus, Susan Brockman, Cella Irvine, Daniel Rowen, David Stiles, Sabina Lanier, and Sue Mingus.

Over the T'ai Chi years, one name stands out—the late Lou Kleinsmith, a great mentor who inspired in me the desire to teach, for he was an outstandingly creative and joyous teacher of the Form.

"Stand like a balance and move like a wheel."

—Wang Chung-Yueh,

The Treatise on T'ai Chi Ch'uan, 1791

PREFACE

T'ai Chi Ch'uan Is . . .

T'ai Chi Ch'uan is an ancient Chinese exercise dating back to A.D. 1100. It comes to us as a technique of moving with knees slightly bent, slowly and continuously, in a series in which each movement grows out of and into the next. These movements were designed to make the body balanced and supple, in order to both defend against an enemy (T'ai Chi is the quintessential martial art) and to prevent disease and increase longevity.

There are five major T'ai Chi forms: Yang, Wu, Ho, Sun, and Chen. My expertise lies in the Yang-style Short Form, which I learned from the revered Grandmaster Cheng Man-ch'ing, who adapted the shortened form from the Yang-style Long Form. The Yang style (either short or long) is the most universally practiced and accepted form today.

The Beginner's Form, laid out in this book, consists of twenty steps: the first third of the Yang-style Short Form. These twenty steps are in no way a shortcut or an abbreviated version of T'ai Chi. They will teach you a new language of movement, and how to relax deeply, achieve spinal alignment, and ultimately, how to release *ch'i*, the energy flow. A sound knowledge of the first third of the form—of its principles and techniques—is key to the mastery of T'ai Chi.

INTRODUCTION

One Sunday morning nearly thirty years ago, I met some friends in New York's Chinatown for a dim sum breakfast. Across from the restaurant on the second floor of a commercial building was a large sign that read "T'ai Chi Ch'uan Association." I wondered what it meant, and a friend at the table said she thought it was some kind of Chinese exercise. Intrepidly, we crossed the street to take a look.

We climbed up a flight of stairs and peeked into the open door of a large room. A Chinese man in black robes was leading a class of thirty or forty people of various ages. I immediately sensed an unfamiliar peacefulness in the room. The students seemed to be doing nothing and yet everything. It was mysteriously subtle.

I signed up for the class. My first memory is of standing in a long line behind the teacher, trying to imitate his movements. They didn't seem particularly complex, but the steps in fact were so exact that—although I was an actress at the time and quite used to adopting and learning new gestures and attitudes—my body could not easily approximate the positions. Why was something apparently so simple so difficult?

When we moved into a step, we had to hold the position while Grand Master Cheng Man-ch'ing, or Professor as he was called, corrected our postures.

He touched various points on my body to tell me with his hand (he didn't speak a word of English) where to release my tension. When he pressed his hand against my chest, I felt a searing sensation, as if a bullet had gone through me. Then suddenly my chest and arms felt lighter, as if all my weight had dropped into my legs—and my legs, grown heavier, felt as if they were rooted in the earth. At the time, it was an odd, almost unsettling sensation. I had no idea where T'ai Chi would take me. But my gut feeling was: This is an extraordinary experience; I am in the right place. My body was saying *yes*.

I wasn't concerned about rushing through to the end of the whole form to see how it came out. I began to enjoy the way each new step interlocked with the next. I left rigorous sessions feeling invigorated rather than exhausted. I remember liking the way my body was beginning to feel. I had more stamina. And I was learning how to hold myself in correct alignment—a wonderful feeling.

Furthermore, unlike other exercises I had known, T'ai Chi demanded constant, acute mental effort, with the result that my mind never drifted and I was never bored. In order to do the T'ai Chi positions, or shapes, my mind had to dictate very subtle directions to my back, legs, arms, and hands. All parts of the body had to move in sync.

The exercise did many things for me. It calmed me down. Distracting thoughts that crowd the head and vitiate one's energy lost their power when I began to focus on moving my body into the exacting balance required by the form. Eventually, I lost all excess weight. Because the form requires the knees to be bent throughout, my stomach and thighs strengthened. I used to get tired after walking a mile or so in the city; now I never tired and began to love walking. I no longer wondered what I had gotten myself into. In fact, I had entered a profound new world—or, to be accurate, a profound old world, which reaches back to China's ancient history.

The ancient Chinese in their earliest written documents reveal a culture engrossed in the ultimate objective of finding a secret to immortality, or at the very least to a very long life. Toward this end, they tried to understand the way the universe pulsated. They studied nature—not to control it, but to learn from it. There is a story, for instance, about the Great Flood in China's earliest history. During the catastrophe, the waters stagnated and infested the land, giving rise to a plague. The emperor at the time divined from this that, likewise, when people stagnate, they will get sick. He ordered all his people to perform a series of exercises called the Great Dances, designed to promote the flow of energy comparable to the never-ending flow of a river.

From the earliest time the Chinese believed that a person's health is inextricably linked to the flow of energy through his or her body. They had people who observed whether whole herbs increased energy to alleviate certain problems. They analyzed the human body and invented postures to cure specific ailments. Each illness had its own exercise. Although they did not do anatomical dissections, because the body was considered sacred, they knew that the heart was the main organ pumping blood in a continuous circular path and that circulation was the vital current.

The concept at the heart of these investigations and the concept at the heart of T'ai Chi Ch'uan has been what the Chinese call *ch'i* (a different word from the *chi* of T'ai Chi Ch'uan, which means "ultimate"). *Ch'i* is the underpinning for everything in existence. The idea of this vital energy is by no means unique to China—the Greeks called it *pneuma*, the Romans called it *spiritus*, and we in the modern West commonly refer to it as the *life force* or our electromagnetic field. The Chinese interpretation of the role of this vital energy in our day-to-day lives was, and is, unique: they believed, and believe today, that when the flow of *ch'i* throughout the body is restricted or blocked, by either mental or physical trauma, illness develops—and that the cure for such illness is to remove the blockage and set the *ch'i* flowing freely again. Acupuncture, for example, is used to unblock the *ch'i*, but the paramount method—paramount not only because it can be self-administered by anyone at any time but because it is prevention as well as cure—is T'ai Chi Ch'uan.

Along with prescribing herbs and performing energy exercises, the Chinese developed deep, slow breathing techniques which often lasted for hours. "The men of old breathed clear down to their heels," it was said. They believed that if a person became tense with worry or grief, the breath would become shallow and constricted and would in turn prevent the blood from circulating effectively. One must calm the mind as well as exercise the body. Body and mind both should be attended to in order to ensure good health.

The Chinese also studied animal behavior for clues to health and longevity. "As a means to long life," said Chuang Tzu, a fourth-century-B.C. philosopher of the Taoist school, "pass some time like a dormant bear." "Imitate the flappings of a duck, the ape's dance, the owl's fixed stare, the tiger's crouch, the pawings of a bear," said others.[1]

In A.D. 300 a surgeon named Hua To developed a series of movements based on the way animals move called the Frolics of the Five Animals (tiger, deer, bear, monkey, and

---

1. Sophia Delza, *T'ai Chi Chuan* (State University of New York Press, 1985), p. 7.

bird).[2] About four hundred years later, the movements were linked into one continuous pattern. This continuity of movement resulted in a deepening of the performer's concentration and strength and was the precursor of T'ai Chi as a form. It is quite extraordinary to note that some of the same names of the postures that evolved from these early imitations of animals are still being used in our form today, such as Phoenix Flaps Its Wings (in today's version, Stork Spreads Its Wings). Other names of the postures, such as Single Whip, derive from ancient martial techniques indicating how the shape is used against an opponent.

Through the centuries China vacillated between periods of warfare and reigns that were essentially peaceful. However, there was constant pressure from potential invaders attempting to seize their lands. The emperor always maintained a standing army, but within each individual temple the monks had to protect themselves (without government help) against the attacks of bandits.

Martial training in each monastery was quite different from that of the army. In the monasteries that training was far more rigorous, subtle, and intense. To learn perfect control of their bodies, minds, and spirits, religious practitioners trained their *ch'i* to a much deeper level than what occurred in the rest of society. This training was integrated into the martial arts forms they used, and these practices and meditations were passed down secretly within the monasteries.

It was in these monasteries, spread throughout the land, that the differing forms of martial arts developed. Two basic schools evolved: the "outer-extrinsic" school of exercise, where muscular action is intense and energy is forcibly produced, and the soft "inner-extrinsic" school, where the action is nonaggressive and yielding. The soft school is the basis of T'ai Chi Ch'uan as we know it today.

The credit for formalizing the soft-style series of exercises into a unified whole belongs to a Taoist monk, Chang San-feng, who was active around A.D. 1100. As the legend goes, Chang San-feng happened to be walking in the woods when he encountered a crane fighting with a snake. The crane was jabbing at the snake with his long beak in straight angular strikes. The snake was able to avoid the crane by changing his shape and position (staying very soft and resilient), slithering away, and then quickly counterattacking while the bird was still committed to its original thrust. The monk gleaned from this that it would be possible for a weaker opponent to overcome a stronger one if he became soft and elusive. He incorporated this lesson into a new, softer version of a martial art and at the same time a health-promoting exercise.

T'ai Chi Ch'uan loosely translates as "the supreme ultimate martial art." *T'ai* means "supreme," *chi* means "ultimate," and *ch'uan* means "fist." While the word *ch'uan* characterizes the martial art aspect of the discipline, the exercise was (and is) equally considered a means to health and longevity.

Integral to T'ai Chi is Taoism, which teaches us to act without forcing, to move in accordance with the flow of nature—to not push, press, or insist. In T'ai Chi, body and mind are deliberately trained not to counter force with force, but instead to move out of

---

2. Ibid.

the way, to evaporate. The force will lose its effect because there is nothing to receive it. A master of T'ai Chi seems to have no bones in his body. If you touch him, he is like a ghost—where has he gone?

If you look at Chinese painting, you'll see that the landscapes are immense, with huge mountains and vast skies, and that people rendered in it are tiny, almost minuscule. The Chinese were in awe of the vastness and mystery of the universe, of nature. By contrast, Western art places man, large, at the center of the canvas, with nature as a backdrop. It's apparent in certain details of early European painting (for example, globes, maps, calipers, telescopes) that the driving force here is man's newfound excitement at discovering how to control nature. The Chinese, on the other hand, with their reverence for nature, sought to merge themselves with it—to conform to the "great reality."

Two major philosophical schools of lasting importance to the Chinese, Taoism and Confucianism, embrace several ideas deeply embedded in the discipline of T'ai Chi Ch'uan. Taoism is a system of thought based on a study of how the universe actually functions—human beings revering and yielding to its unfathomable mysteries, to be in harmony with, not in rebellion against, the fundamental laws of nature. Confucianism, on the other hand, is a system teaching right conduct—the cultivation of uprightness in order to live a calm and ordered life in cooperation with all others in society.

T'ai Chi Ch'uan requires the practitioner to be nonaggressive in action (Taoism) and to maintain steady, calm, and precise control of the actions of the form (Confucianism).

T'ai Chi Ch'uan is as old as these great philosophies; its roots reach back twenty-three centuries. Like a great classic in literature that has lasted because it has withstood the test of time, T'ai Chi Ch'uan has for centuries been the exercise of choice for millions of Chinese, who every day at dawn and at dusk go to their parks in the cities and countryside and engage in this rhythmical, ballet-like exercise in order to center themselves and feel invigorated. They have been doing this for hundreds of years—the young, the old, and the very old. T'ai Chi Ch'uan is unique in its ability to be embraced by everyone of all ages and physical abilities.

T'ai Chi requires no special equipment. All you need are clothes loose-fitting enough to allow you to move freely and flat shoes with soles that won't stick to the floor. It can be practiced in a space of no more than four or five feet. And it can be done in a period of ten minutes or less, at any time of day, though preferably upon rising, when it will invigorate and center you. As Grand Master Cheng Man-ching said, morning is the best time to swallow the Ch'i of Heaven. When possible, do the form again the last thing in the evening before you go to bed, so that its soft, fluid movements will dissolve the fatigue and stresses of the day. T'ai Chi is "stress management" at its most classic and elegant.

For all its practical advantages, T'ai Chi's chief attraction for new devotees stems primarily from the extraordinary beauty of the form—its incarnation of total peacefulness.

THE PRINCIPLES

In T'ai Chi, mind and body achieve, ideally, complete coordination. This mind-body harmony is the premise from which the principles of T'ai Chi derive. The bodily movements are the principles in action. These eight principles, as I teach them in my classes, are: Alignment, Relaxation, Slowness, Continuity, Circularity, Polarity, Concentration, and Centering.

Alignment

Although T'ai Chi is performed with the knees slightly bent, the torso must have a plumb-line straightness, from the top of the head to the base of the spine, for it is this perfect spinal alignment that allows the *ch'i*—the life energy—to flow effortlessly through the body.

In thinking of your own alignment (or lack of it) it may be helpful to visualize a set of children's building blocks, piled one on top of another, and to remember that if one of the blocks is pushed even slightly out of place, the entire column will wobble or fall down.

Of course, though our own building blocks—our head, neck, chest, pelvis, thighs, and feet—are not very likely to be in a straight line, that doesn't mean we will necessarily wobble or fall. For no matter how out of alignment we may be, we have, from childhood on, learned to hold ourselves upright and keep our balance by unconsciously tightening certain muscles and tendons. Unfortunately, this tightening that helps hold us in place not only is a hidden drain on our energy but also can inhibit the free and healthful flow of blood and oxygen through our body.

T'ai Chi will, among other things, adjust you to your true and central line of balance. And, in time, this adjustment, with all its energy-enhancing benefits, will become natural and permanent. Meanwhile, it is essential, before you take your first step in T'ai Chi, to put yourself as best you can into alignment. Stand with your feet shoulder-distance apart, keeping the knees slightly bent. Now . . .

Straighten the head. Imagine that your head is suspended at the crown by a string from the ceiling. Your eyes are level, looking straight ahead; your nose is lined up directly over your navel; your tongue is resting on the upper palate behind the front teeth.

Soften the chin. Lower it and gently pull it in. If the chin is the least bit thrust out, and you try to balance a book on your head, the book will fall. While the action of lifting the head and softening and pulling in the chin may be uncomfortable at first, it will straighten the neck, the cervical region of the spine that is crucial to proper alignment.

Drape the shoulders. Your arms and hands are by your sides. If they are behind you, your chest will pop out; if they are in front of you, you will be round-shouldered.

Sink the chest. To sink the chest properly, take a large inhale of breath, then exhale slowly as if air were seeping out of a balloon. At the same time, drop your rib cage and you will feel your center of gravity move from the upper body to the lower body. You are now weighted correctly—light on top, heavy at the base. As you inhale again, think of the breath as traveling from the base of the spine up each vertebra to the top of your head. Then exhale down the channel of the back. When you are practicing this, press your chest down with your hand as you slowly inhale and exhale to make sure your chest doesn't rise.

Drop the tailbone. Place your hand on the base of your spine. Now gently push the tailbone forward and down, without tensing your buttocks. If this is done correctly, the small of your back will fill out. To maintain a straight spine, picture a rope attached to the tailbone: at the other end of the rope is a ten-thousand-pound weight pulling the tailbone down.

Open the joints. Because T'ai Chi usually requires you to balance most of your weight on one leg or the other, the tendency is to tighten and tense the muscles around the joints—particularly the knees and ankles—in order to hold a position. As you practice, two things will help eliminate this tension. First, your legs will naturally become stronger. Second, through realignment, you will discover your center of gravity, the central line of balance, which will enable you to be so truly stabilized, with one leg or the other solidly rooted to the ground, that you can release the hold on the joints.

All movements and positions should be explored with a sense of bodily looseness. You must never move into any posture with rigidity. Think of the movements of a mime, who is a master of control, yet always fluid and pliant.

Here is a quick review of the key posture points:
- Head suspended by a string from above
- Eyes level
- Nose over navel
- Tongue on upper palate behind front teeth
- Chin in
- Chest deflated
- Arms at your sides
- Tailbone dropped
- Joints open
- Feet planted firmly on the ground

Relaxation

Relaxation as it is understood in T'ai Chi means getting rid of the body's rigidities and the mind's resistances. The method I use for learning to relax is a kind of dialogue in which the mind talks to the body and the body talks to the mind. The key words of this dialogue are: *sink, melt, let go, drop.*

For instance, if you are worried, the muscles of your *forehead* will be pulled tight. Tell the forehead to let go and feel the frown loosen. This physical loosening is, in turn, the body's way of telling the mind to let go of its worry.

Feel your *shoulders*. If they are tight, tell them to sink and melt. To understand the feeling of relaxed shoulders, lift them up to your ears, then let them drop. This has a calming effect on the mind that is similar to the common act of pausing and taking a deep breath. But because it is more physical its message to the mind is more convincing.

Is your *chest* hard and tense? It is probably puffed out, Marine Corps style, in a way that makes your body top-heavy and forces you unknowingly to tense your muscles to stay in balance. Let your rib cage drop. Remember that your true center of strength is not in your chest but in your gut—one and a third inches below your navel in the area the Chinese call the *tan-tien*.

The *pelvis* is another area of often unexpected rigidity. Put your hand on your hip-bone and bend your knees a bit. Now tell your hipbone to let go, to soften. It will be difficult at first to feel whether this is happening, but in time you will be able to discern where your skeletal structure and muscle systems are taut, and you will learn to direct your mind to each place in your body to evaporate the tension.

As you learn the patterns of the form, your *legs* will be moving into positions you don't normally use. You may feel rigid as you attempt the shapes. Touch your thigh and calf muscles and check for tightness. Melt the tension in the leg that is carrying most of the weight; your other leg should now feel like a rag doll's. As you shift your weight from one leg to the other, the tendency is to clench the thigh muscle that is going to bear the weight. But the shifting of weight should never be done that way—rather, feel the transfer of weight as a "giving up" to gravity, a letting go, not a pressing down. With your mind constantly directing it, your weight will sink more and more into the base of your feet, which are rooted in the earth.

Above all, to relax means to remove all mental as well as physical resistances. As disturbances beset the mind, you must learn not to fight them, but simply to let them come and go. As your philosophical understanding of T'ai Chi deepens, you will be putting into practice the profound doctrine of nonresistance that lies at the heart of what has been called "this great system of human betterment."

Slowness

T'ai Chi has a mysterious beauty. The practitioners move slowly, as if they are immersed in water from the neck down. If you've ever run down the beach and into the ocean, you've felt the sudden resistance of the water change your speed. You must slow up. Actually, you yield to the pressure all around you and let the water in a sense guide your movements. This shifting of concentration, away from your own personal being to heightened awareness and connection with nature, gives the person doing the form a look of intense yet sublime focus.

The slowness that occurs from moving through imaginary water allows you time to achieve the impeccable balance required of each shape. Further, by experiencing the air as heavy, like ocean water, one feels lighter, more buoyant. You are striving for that lightness, since the aim of T'ai Chi is to eliminate hardness in the body and to become supple and pliant like seaweed.

Continuity

Hand in hand with the principle of slowness is the principle of continuity. T'ai Chi should be done at one slow, steady speed, without any interruption. This requires diligent concentration. Be careful not to dismiss certain transitions between moves as so brief and inconsequential that you can rush through them. In T'ai Chi, every beat of every step, no matter how small it may seem, is carried out with equal respect and attention. To understand the concept of continuity, the Chinese like to picture reeling silk from the cocoon of a silkworm. The thread must be pulled very slowly and steadily—if it is jerked suddenly, it will break. The thread will also break if it is slackened and then pulled again. Think of the form as one continuous delicate pulling of the thread.

A natural tendency for the beginner is to come to a complete stop between postures. Instead, keep the movement going. As you reach the peak of one posture, be ready to melt into the next, like the dip and swell of ocean waves.

Circularity

T'ai Chi is performed circularly. Its movements are a continuous flow of circles, arcs, ovals, spirals, undulations. There are no angles, edges, or straight lines. Imagine a Ping-Pong ball floating on top of the water. If you were to try pushing the ball under the water, it would slip away, turning circularly. As you flow and undulate, there is nothing for your opponent (thinking for a moment of T'ai Chi as the supreme defensive martial art) to grab onto and control. It is worth noting again that many of the steps of T'ai Chi still retain their original martial art names. However, T'ai Chi as a system of self-defense need not concern you at this stage, if it ever does. Beyond martial arts, these light, airy, circular movements will keep your muscles properly toned and will, as the very name of this principle implies, improve your circulation. And they will be particularly helpful to those with arthritic-like joint problems. Practiced regularly, these soft and rounded movements are the best way in the world to stay loose.

Polarity

T'ai Chi organically expresses the Chinese philosophy of yin and yang—the positive (yang) and negative (yin) forces of the universe: If there is sky, there must be earth; if there is day, there must be night; if there is up, there must be down. The moves in T'ai Chi embody this basic polarity of existence. If you turn to the right, you then turn to the left; when the right leg is "full" (with all the body's weight resting on it), the left leg is "empty" or "hollow," and vice versa.

Such shifts are never abrupt. For example, as you shift your weight from the full leg into the empty one, think of an old-fashioned three-minute egg timer, with the sand sifting slowing from top to bottom. Now imagine your empty leg, after you've placed it on the ground, slowly filling up with sand until a sense of weight and fullness is achieved and the opposite leg has become hollow. It is always with this "hollow leg" that you will step (whether forward, sideward, or backward), and you will "step empty"—like a cat with soft pads. Only after the hollow leg is resting on the ground do you shift your weight.

Be careful, too, not to lead with your hipbone. In this as in all the moves, no part of the body should jut out. Remember that in T'ai Chi, polarity is what is unified and made one.

Concentration

While the body is loose, with movements as fluid and pliant as those of a mime, the mind must be at every instant alert and focused. All moves in T'ai Chi are made consciously. The attention required to do this is as exacting as, for instance, putting a golf ball into a hole. The slightest mental distraction, the slightest lack of alignment, sends the ball off course. With your mind engaged, you are able to get closer and closer to the perfection of the form. T'ai Chi is a meditation in movement in which the very preciseness of the individual movements themselves concentrates the mind and clears it of extraneous thoughts.

Centering

In the philosophy of T'ai Chi, the *ch'i* cannot move itself but must always be awakened, moved, and directed by the power of the mind. And where the mind directs the *ch'i* first of all is to the true center of the body, the *tan-tien*, located one and a third inches below the navel. All movement in T'ai Chi is initiated from the *tan-tien*. This may be hard to understand at first, but imagine you have a belt on your hips with a rope attached to the buckle (the area of the *tan-tien*) that is pulling you forward. As you move through the form, it is your concentration on the *tan-tien* (the presence and pull of this belt buckle) that centers you. Eventually, the *ch'i* power accumulates in the *tan-tien* and can be directed by the mind to any part of the body.

THE 70/30 POSTURE

The essential stance in T'ai Chi is the 70/30 Posture and is repeated throughout the form. It is called the 70/30 Posture because the front foot holds 70 percent of your weight while the back foot holds 30 percent.

The posture is awkward at first, since your body is not used to shaping itself this way, and should be practiced, on both the right and the left sides, before proceeding to the beginning of the form.

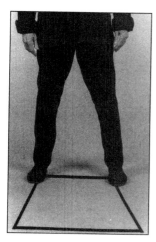

1. Stand with your feet parallel and shoulder width apart. Now, with your imagination, project a rectangle on the ground in front of you. Imagine that you are standing on the two back corners of the short side of the rectangle.

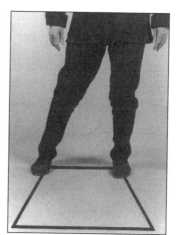

2. Put all of your weight onto the foot that will be placed in the forward position—in this case, the left foot.

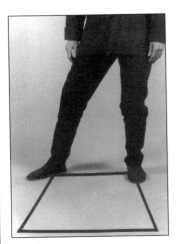

3. Now pick up the toes of the empty right foot (empty because your weight is on the left) and pivot on the right heel so that the toes turn to a 45-degree angle.

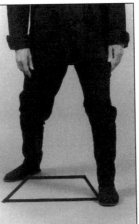

6. Shift 70 percent of your weight into your front leg; feel the weight in the thigh, not the knee. Bend your knees. Drop your pelvis down slightly in that posture (without sticking your buttocks out), as if you were settling onto the saddle of a horse. Make sure you are sitting in the center of the saddle, not on the horse's neck or rump. Relax and drop the right knee to loosen it so that it feels almost empty. You are now in the 70/30 stance.

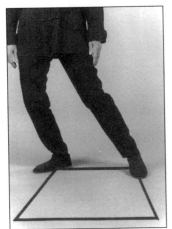

4. Shift all of your weight into your right foot until the heel of the left foot releases (lifts from the ground).

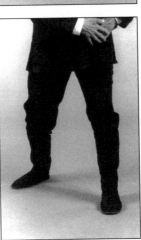

7. Sink your left hip—which will root you even further into this shape.

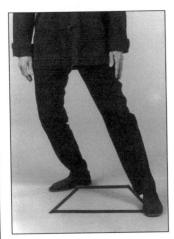

5. Pick the left foot slightly off the ground and, moving it in an absolutely straight line, place it directly in the front left corner of the imaginary rectangle, the heel touching first. If you have to lean to get there, you are stepping out too far.

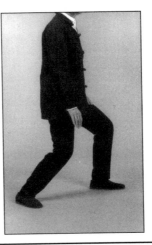

8. When you settle your body into the 70/30 Posture, the left knee should not go beyond the toes. The lower part of the left leg, from the knee to the foot, forms a straight line.

Please note: Whenever you execute the 70/30 stance, be sure you arrive in the position with your feet shoulder-distance apart. Otherwise you will not be able to get your body to sink between your legs.

Now begin again, this time moving the right leg into the front position of the rectangle.

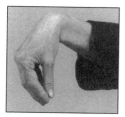

HAND POSITIONS

Bird's Beak

In T'ai Chi, you never want to sever the unity between hand and wrist, except in this one design, in which you form your hand into the shape of a bird's beak. In this position, the fingers and thumb come together as if pinching salt. The middle finger is furthest out. Fingers are not clutched, but held loosely. See p. 62, Position 5.

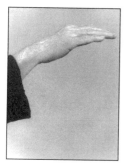

Swan's Head

In this shape, sometimes called Beautiful Lady's Hand, bring the thumb next to the index finger. All five digits become one unit, close together but not squeezed tight (a piece of paper could slip through each finger).

The forearm, from the elbow to the tip of the middle finger, forms a slight curve, as if the arm is resting on a silken pillow.

For Swan's Head, first concentrate on the hang of the elbow and then gradually extend your arm, "seeking the straight in the curve." See p. 66, Position 9.

BREATHING

When practicing the form, breathe naturally through the nose with your mouth closed. Do not worry about when to inhale or exhale. Concentrating on breathing at this early stage can put too much of a burden on you; forcing the breath will cause tension. In advanced training, you will coordinate deep diaphragmatic breathing with every posture of the form, but that is after you've understood the steps and assimilated the principles.

THE FLOOR PATTERN

Because the positioning in T'ai Chi is so precise, instructions for placement of the feet and body are often given with specific compass directions.

When you begin your practice, position yourself facing a flat wall or, if outdoors, a space that is clearly defined. The side of the room or space you face becomes "imaginary north." With that determined, the right side of the room is east, the left side of the room is west, and behind you is south. Likewise, the right front corner is northeast, and the left front corner is northwest; the back right corner is southeast, and the back left corner is southwest.

In this book, each posture is presented both from the front and from the back (as if you are practicing behind a teacher) or in some instances, for clarity, the side.

THE POSTURES

POSTURE 1 — PREPARATION

POSITION 1

Stand with your heels together, feet in the shape of a V. Imagine that your head is suspended by a string from above. Eyes are level, chin is soft and in. Chest is deflated, tailbone down, arms draped at your sides, knees and ankles unlocked. Relax.

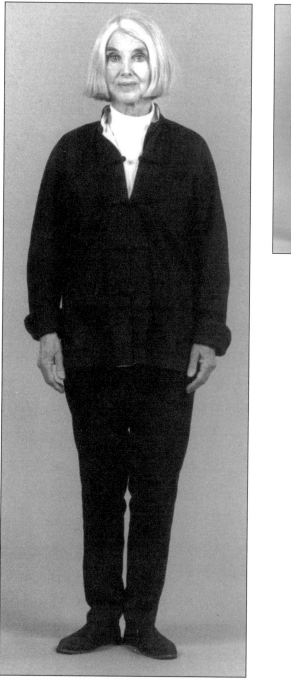

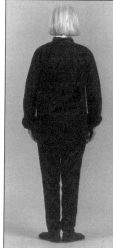

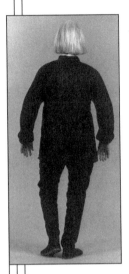

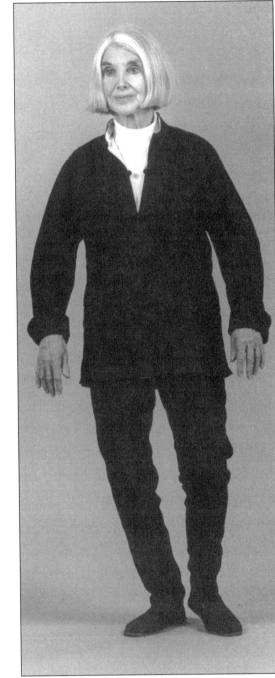

POSITION 2

Bend your knees slightly. Like an old-fashioned egg timer (in which the sand gradually flows from the top to the bottom), imagine the sand pouring down the right leg until the heel of your left foot releases. As you do this, turn the back of the wrists so that they face front (north). Do not lean to the right when you shift the weight, but maintain a perpendicular balance.

POSITION 3

Balanced on your right leg, step out with your left foot (empty of weight), keeping it low to the ground, and place the foot, facing straight ahead, under your left shoulder. To accomplish this move, your body will turn the slightest bit to the right, but do not lean to the right. Stay aligned.

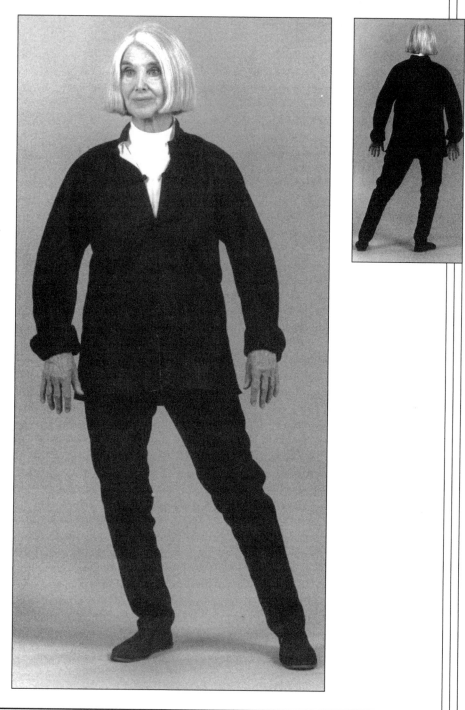

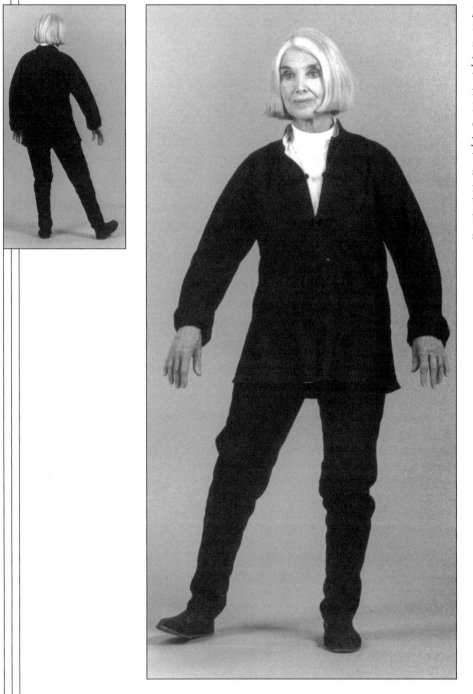

POSITION 4
Slowly pour the sand down into your left leg. The toes of your right foot will release. Keep both knees equally bent as you do this. The tendency is to straighten the right leg as you bring up the toes, but both knees stay bent.

POSITION 5

Turn slightly to the left to straighten your right foot, keeping your knees bent. Do not turn from the groin so that the leg "separates" from the torso, but turn from the hip, which will keep the torso and the leg as a single unit.

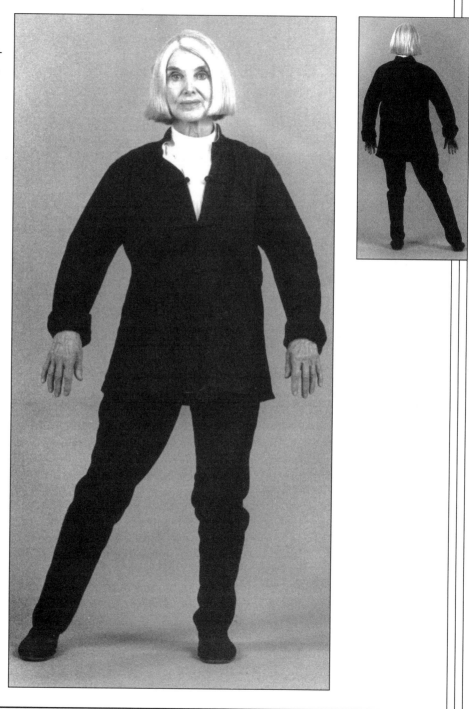

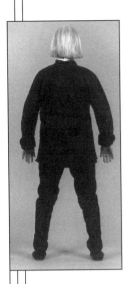

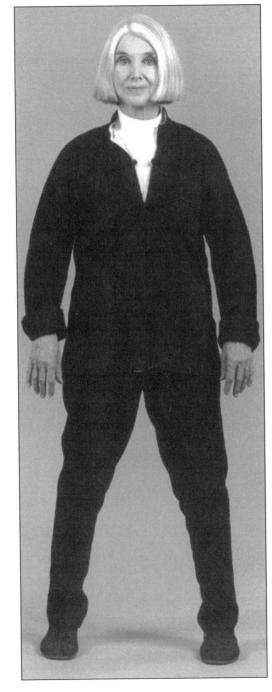

POSITION 6

Shift your weight into your right thigh. Your thighs will become equally heavy. Imagine that your head is attached to a string from the ceiling; the string pulls you slowly upward until you're standing straight, knees unlocked. Your feet are parallel, shoulder distance apart, and the toes lined up.

Posture 2 — BEGINNING

Position 1

Imagine that you have a puppet string attached to the back of each wrist. Let the puppet strings bring the backs of the wrists slowly up to the shoulder level. It should take little effort to do this, since you are barely using your muscles to raise your arms. Your elbows are slightly bent, pointing to the ground; fingers are dangling down. Be sure not to lift your shoulders as you raise your arms.

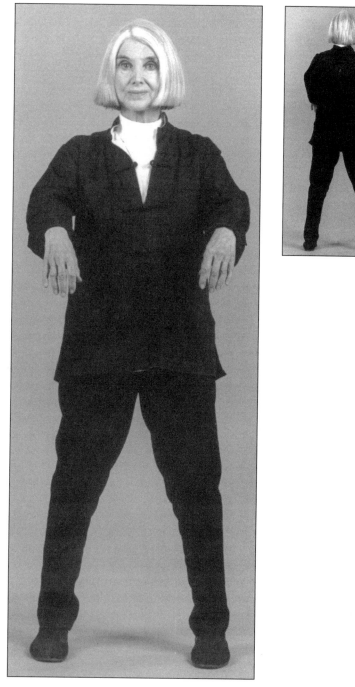

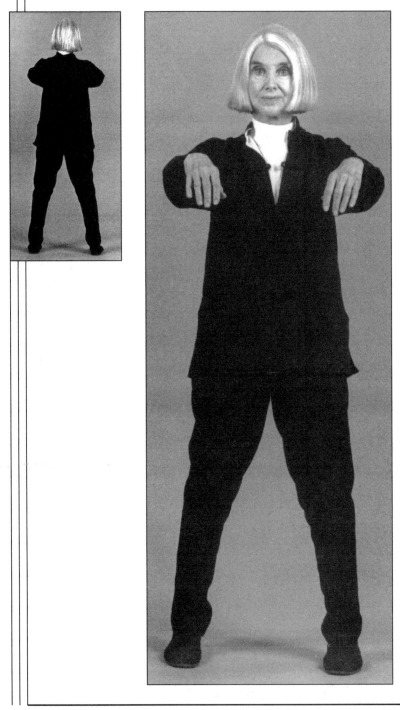

POSITION 2

Your arms arrive at shoulder
level, your fingers dangling
loosely; elbows are still pointing to the ground. You have a
nice extension but not so that
your elbows lock. If you were
to place a flat board from
your shoulder to your wrist,
it would rest perfectly hori-
zontally.

POSITION 3

Extend your fingers so that it feels as if your arms and hands are resting on ocean water. You should feel a floating sensation as if your arms are being supported by the buoyancy of the water.

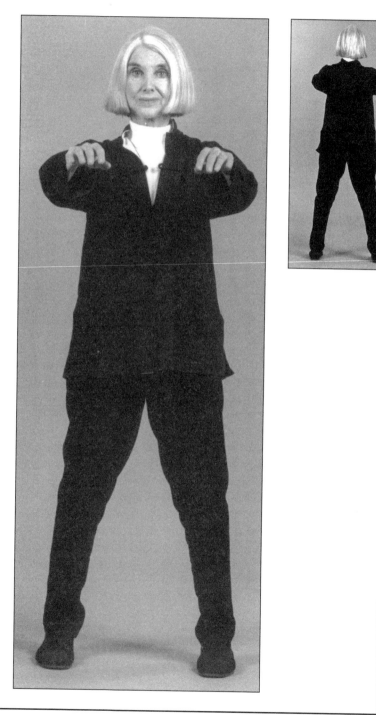

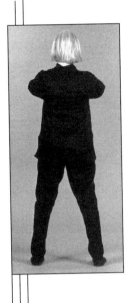

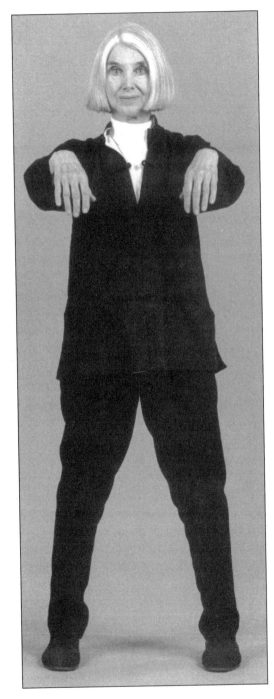

POSITION 4

Drop your hands, fingers loose. Bend your elbows as you bring the wrists slowly, in a straight path, back to the shoulders. Imagine, as you bring the wrists back, that you have sand in each wrist and that the sand is sifting down into the elbows.

POSITION 5

Elbows feel very heavy.
The wrists come all the
way back to the shoul-
ders. Imagine you are
underwater from the
neck down.

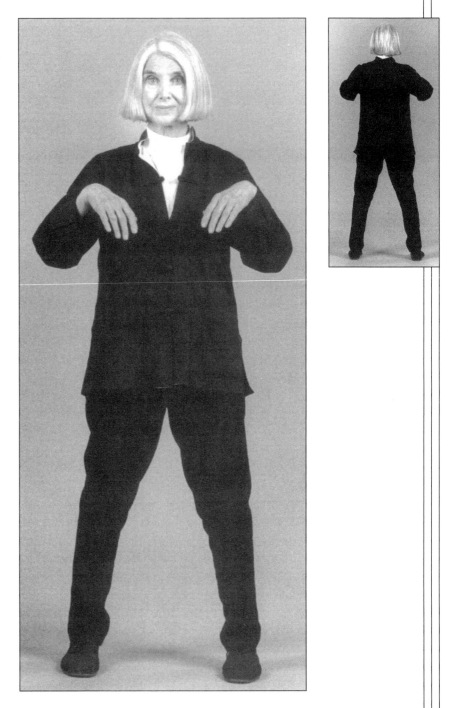

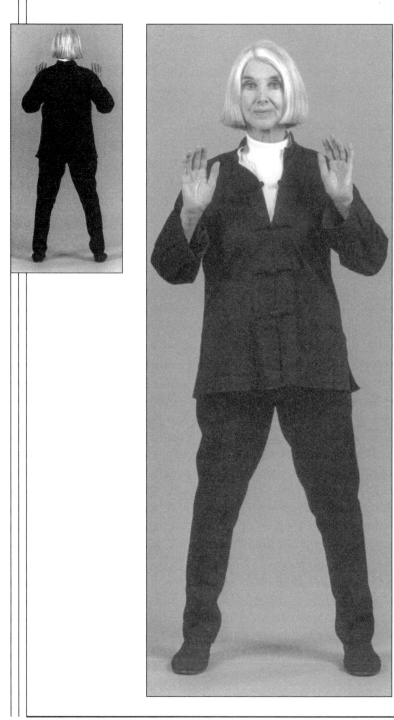

POSITION 6
Your fingers float up to the surface of the water.

POSITION 7

Your arms descend as, with the heels of the palms leading, you push down through water. Imagine now that the sand in the elbows is pouring down into the fingertips as your hands float downward.

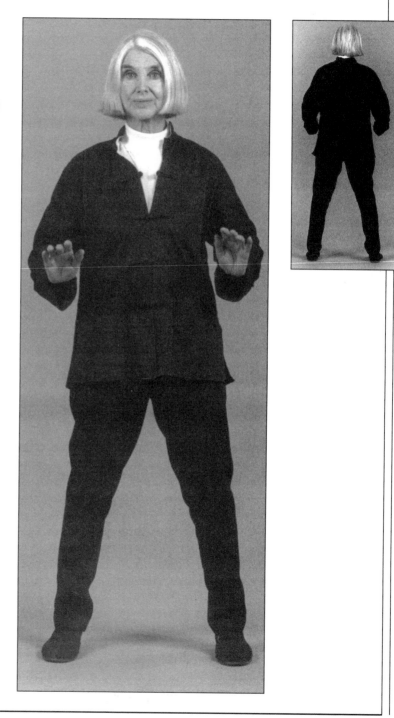

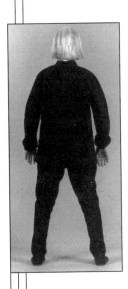

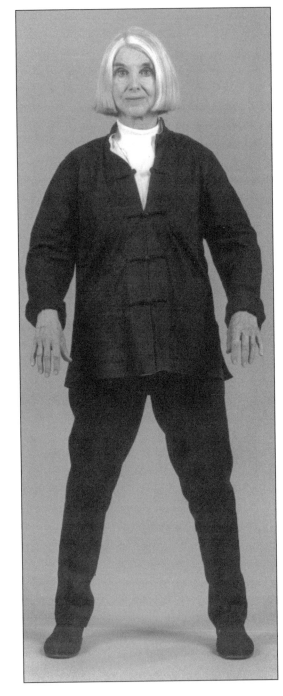

POSITION 8

Your palms are now at your sides, still sensing the density of the water. Don't let them become dead weight. Chest is deflated, shoulders are relaxed, elbows and knees unlocked, joints open.

POSTURE 3 — GRASP SPARROW'S TAIL, WARD OFF, LEFT

POSITION 1
Bend your knees slightly. Shift 100 percent of your weight into your left leg. From this point on, both knees stay quarter-bent throughout the entire exercise.

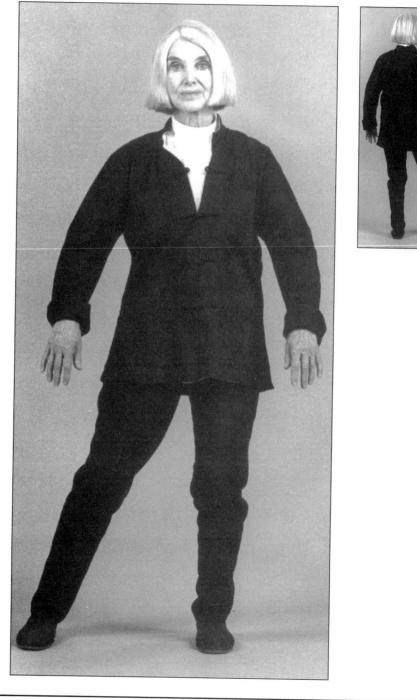

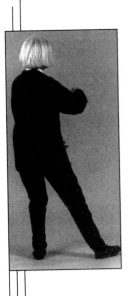

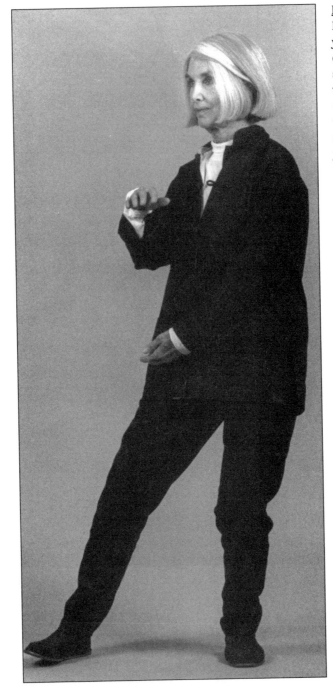

POSITION 2

Release the toes of your right foot, pivot on the heel, and slowly turn your waist to the right (east). At the same time, in the same slow rhythm, raise your right hand to the level of your armpit, palm down, and your left hand to your pelvic bone, directly under the other hand, palm up. Imagine you are holding a beach ball. No clutching or tensing.

POSITION 3

You are now facing directly toward the right wall (east). All of your weight is in your left leg; your right leg is empty, toes off the ground. Head is suspended by a string from above; chest is sunk, tailbone dropped. You are completely relaxed.

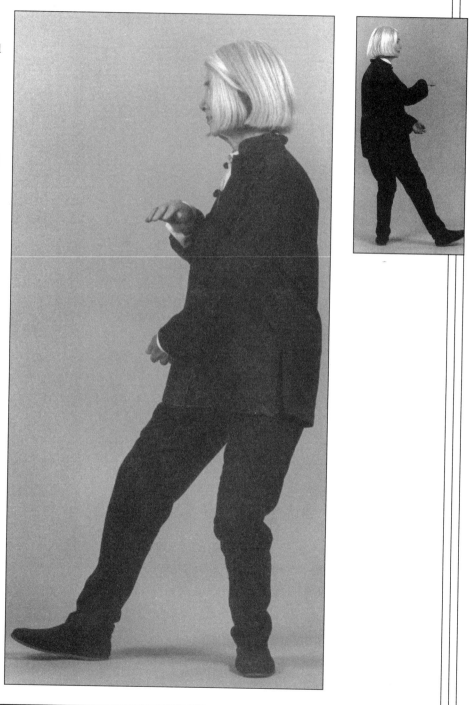

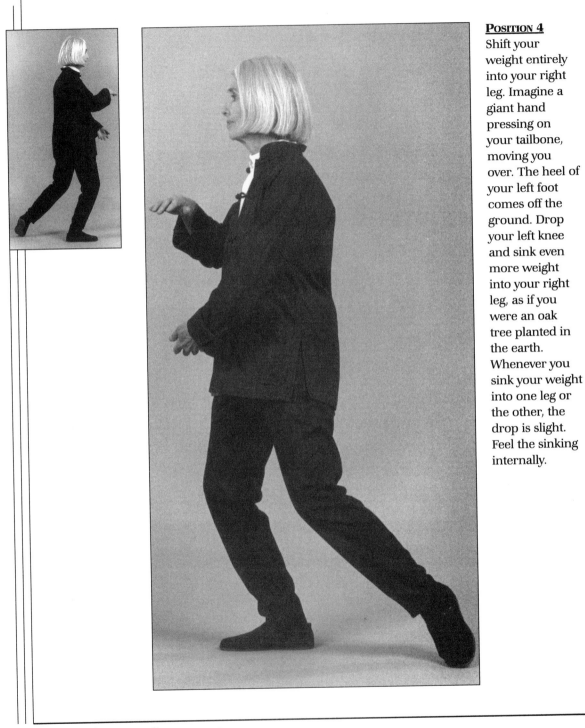

POSITION 4
Shift your weight entirely into your right leg. Imagine a giant hand pressing on your tailbone, moving you over. The heel of your left foot comes off the ground. Drop your left knee and sink even more weight into your right leg, as if you were an oak tree planted in the earth. Whenever you sink your weight into one leg or the other, the drop is slight. Feel the sinking internally.

POSITION 5
Turn to face
the front right
corner (north-
east). As you
turn, you will
feel more of
your weight
sink down into
your right leg.

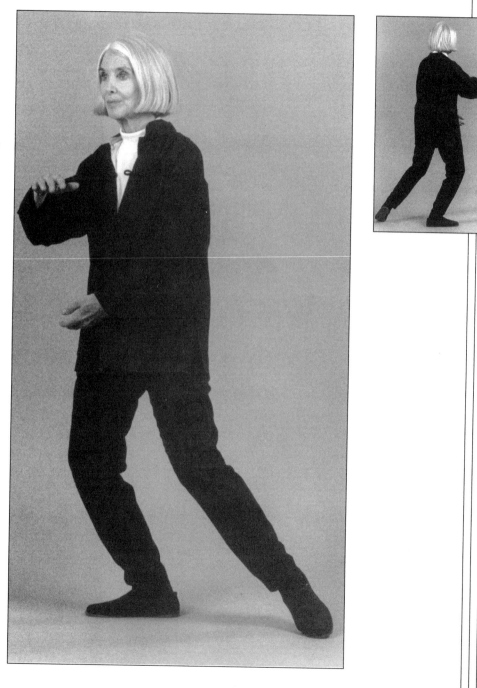

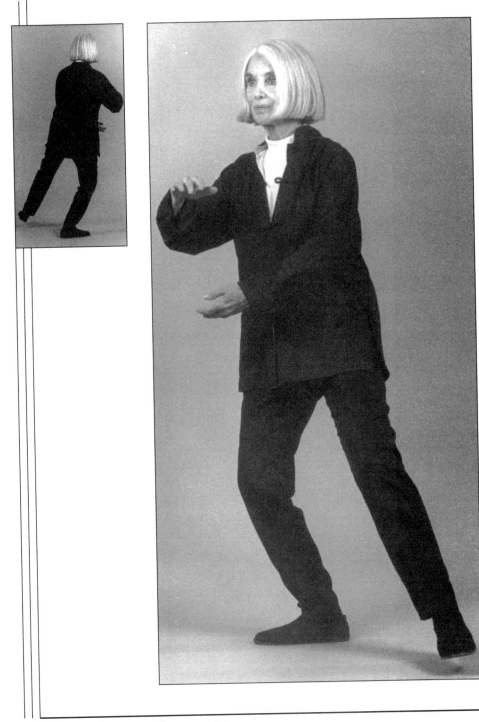

POSITION 6

Balanced and rooted in your right leg, take one step forward with your left foot, the heel touching first (north). Set the left foot down empty; do not bear any of your weight on this foot. Avoid the tendency to lean as you lift your left leg to step out; keep the leg low to the ground and do not overextend it.

POSITION 7

Gradually start shifting most of your weight into your empty left leg. It is important that you stay facing the corner as you make this shift. Keep both knees equally bent.

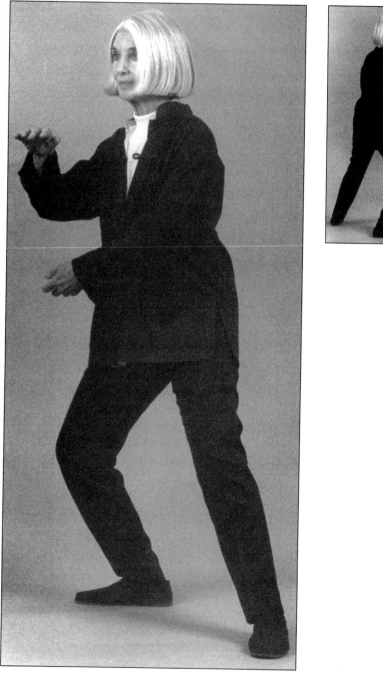

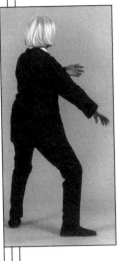

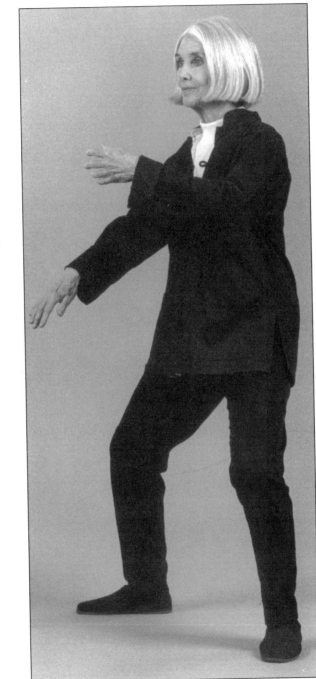

Position 8

You will feel a heaviness in your left thigh as your right thigh lightens. The upper body is completely relaxed, chest sunk, tailbone down. Simultaneously with the leg shift, your hands pass each other. Your right hand (heel of the palm leading) gently pushes down through the ocean water as your left hand rises up in an arc in front of your body to protect your chest. Keep your elbows down, pointing to the ground; arms are fluid and light, empty of tension.

POSITION 9

When 70 percent of your weight is in your left leg, pick up the toes of your right foot and pivot on the heel. Turn your waist to the front (north) while bringing your hip, leg, and right foot around to a 45-degree angle. Always keep the back leg bent as you bring your toes around. Don't get into the habit of straightening and bending again.

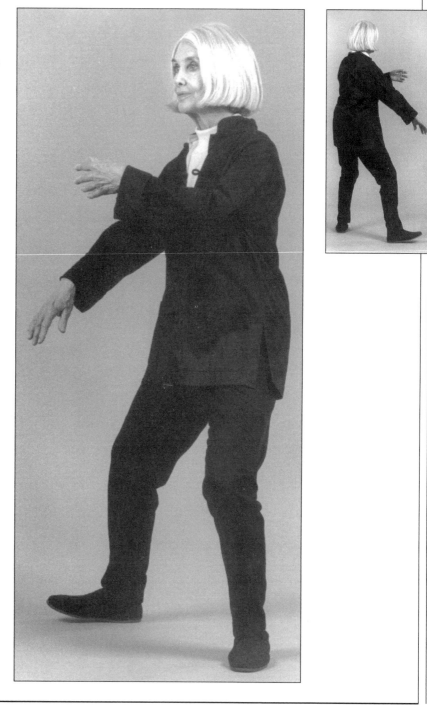

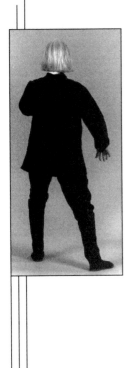

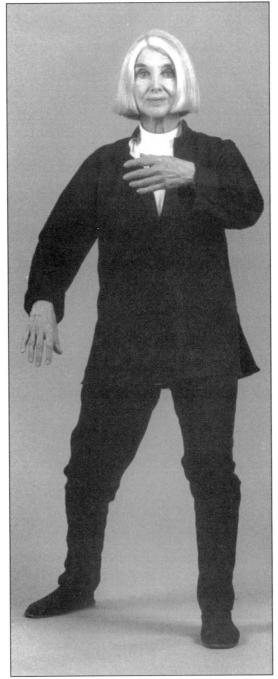

POSITION 10

You have assumed the 70/30 Posture—70 percent of your weight is in your left leg and 30 percent is in your right leg. Your pelvic bones are facing directly front (north). The forward knee is perpendicular to the ground. Without stopping the momentum, relax in this stance by dropping your hips as if you are sitting on the saddle of a horse. But remember, this does not mean you bend more. Let go inwardly.

Posture 4 — GRASP SPARROW'S TAIL, WARD OFF, RIGHT

Position 1

Continuing from the previous position (the 70/30 stance), push your tailbone forward and shift 100 percent of your weight into your left leg. Move from the base of your spine so you don't lean forward. As you do this, turn your left palm over, keeping it where it is, and bring your right palm underneath to create another beach ball—palm sees palm. The heel of your right foot releases, and your right knee drops. The right leg is now completely hollow. Keep loose and relaxed.

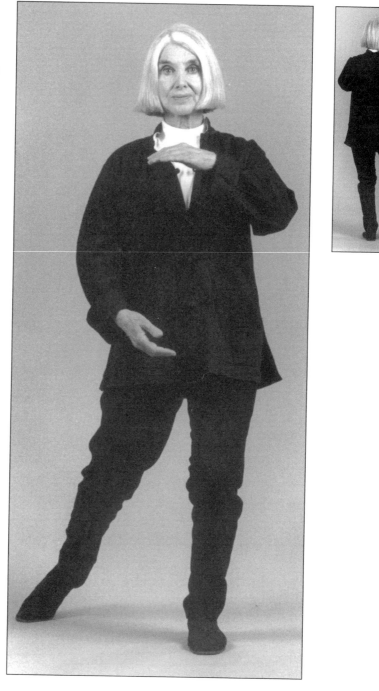

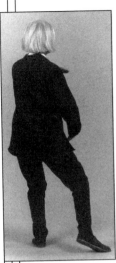

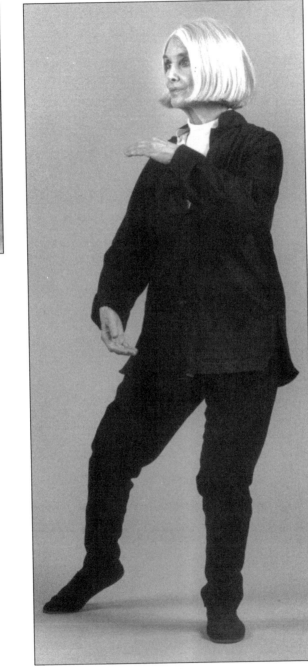

POSITION 2

Turn right and face the front right corner (northeast) again. Keep holding the beach ball, very lightly, elbows down. Sink the weight of your left leg even deeper into the ground in order to ensure your balance.

POSITION 3

Step out with your right foot, aiming for the right-hand corner of an imaginary rectangle projected directly toward the right wall (east). Keep the foot low to the ground so you don't tense your upper body as you step.

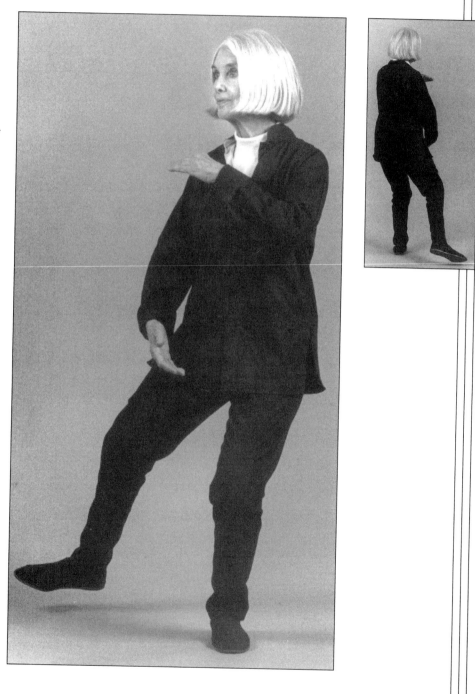

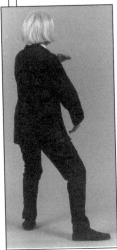

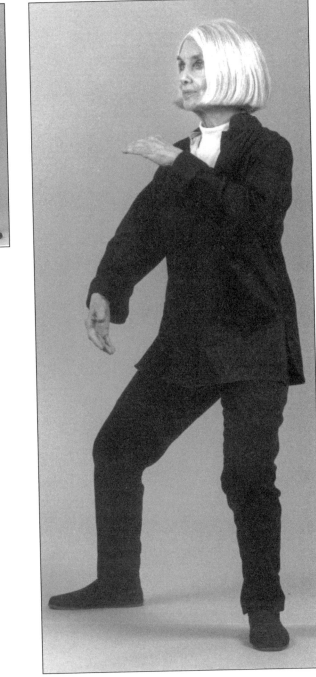

POSITION 4

Place the right heel where the toe was, without putting any weight on it. Think of it as hollow. Make sure that you have a wide enough stance (shoulder distance) as you place the foot, and that the foot points directly to the right wall (east). You are still facing the corner (northeast).

POSITION 5

Slowly shift 70 percent of your weight into your empty right leg. Keep your left palm where it is. In unison with the shift, let the right palm (facing in) slowly rise directly in front of your body, out and up in an arc, elbow down and relaxed, until it reaches the front of your chest. Keep your nose over your navel during the move so that your head continues to face the front corner (northeast).

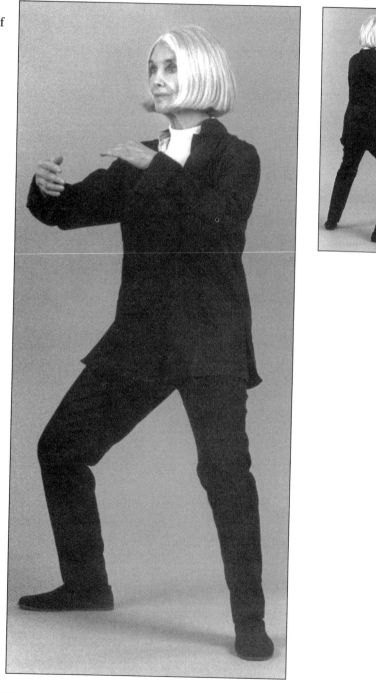

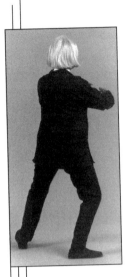

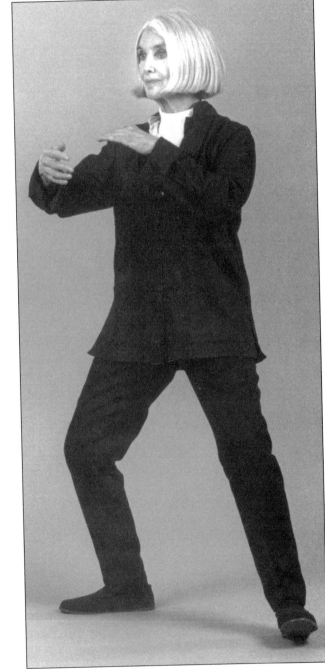

POSITION 6

When 70 percent of your weight has gone into your right thigh, release the toes of your left foot, in order to make the turn to the right wall. The release of the back (in this case, left) foot is like unhinging a gate. Lifting the toes, or "unhinging the gate," makes it possible to turn the body.

POSITION 7

Pivot on your left heel as you turn your waist while bringing your hip, leg, and left foot around to a 45-degree angle to face directly to the right wall (east). Your left foot is now at a 45-degree angle. The left palm comes along with the turn (it does not move itself), and at the last moment, by dropping your left elbow a bit more, the fingers direct themselves behind the thumb of the right hand. You are now in the 70/30 Posture—70 percent of your weight is in your right leg and 30 percent is in your left leg. Relax.

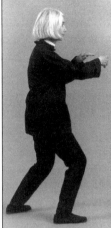

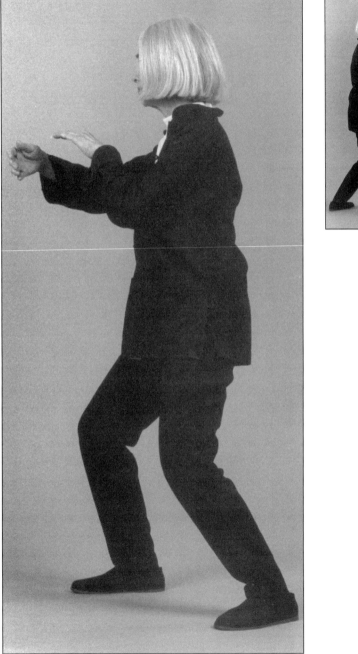

POSTURE 5 — GRASP SPARROW'S TAIL, ROLL BACK

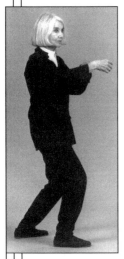

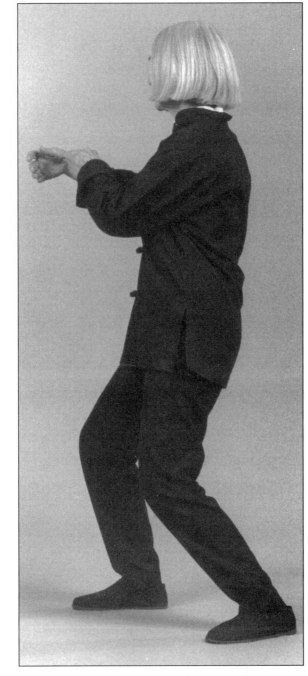

POSITION 1
Without interrupting the momentum, keep your weight in the 70/30 stance and turn your navel toward the back right corner (southeast). Think of melting and dropping your right hipbone in order to rotate your hips, shoulders, and head into this position. Your right leg will feel even heavier with the turn.

POSITION 2

Now shift all of your weight into your left leg, as if you are sitting down on a straight-back chair. Carry the whole upper body as one unit. You are facing directly to the right wall (east) again. As you sit back, your left hand drops under your right elbow, palm up. At the same time, your right elbow bends as your right forearm rises, palm facing north.

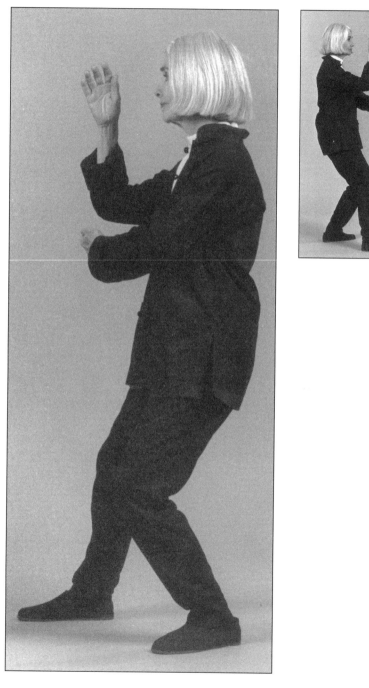

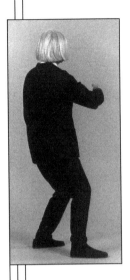

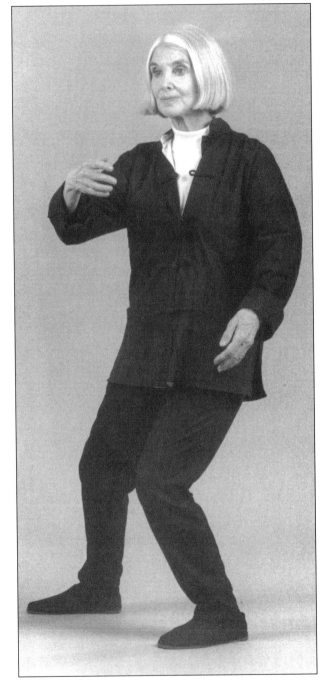

Melt your left hip-bone as you start rotating your waist to the front (north). Keep all of your weight on your left leg. Don't move your right foot with the turn; it rests flat on the floor, empty. Because of the momentum of the turn, your left arm drops slowly down to where the 6 would be on the face of a clock. At the same time, your right arm moves with your body as it turns, and is now protecting your chest.

POSITION 4
Continue
rotating to
the front
(north),
bringing the
left arm
slowly up to
9 on the
clock.
Imagine that
the arm is
being lifted
by a puppet
string at the
wrist; the
shoulder is
dropped,
elbow loose,
forearm
empty of
tension.

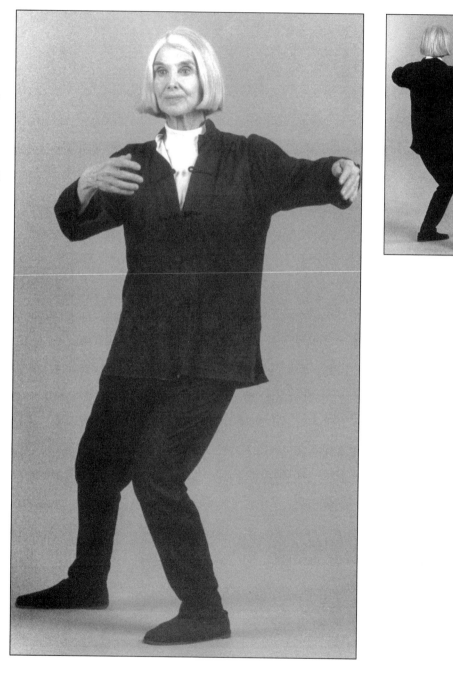

POSTURE 6 — GRASP SPARROW'S TAIL, PRESS

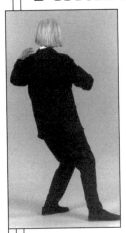

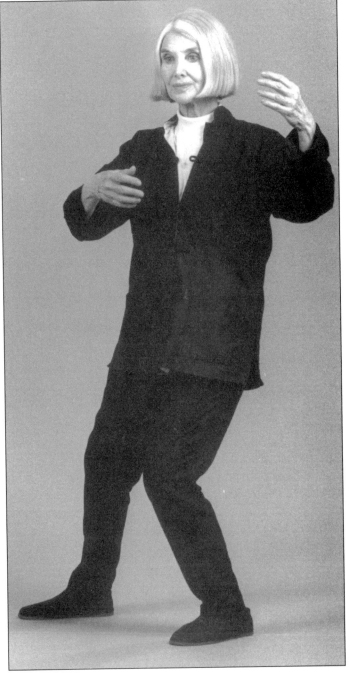

POSITION 1
As you begin to shift the weight back into the right leg, release the left elbow so it sinks even more and the left hand circles up to just under the earlobe.

POSITION 2

Keep the left arm close to the body and moving with you as you shift 70 percent of your weight into your right leg. The right palm continues to protect your chest. The left palm is moved by the shift forward.

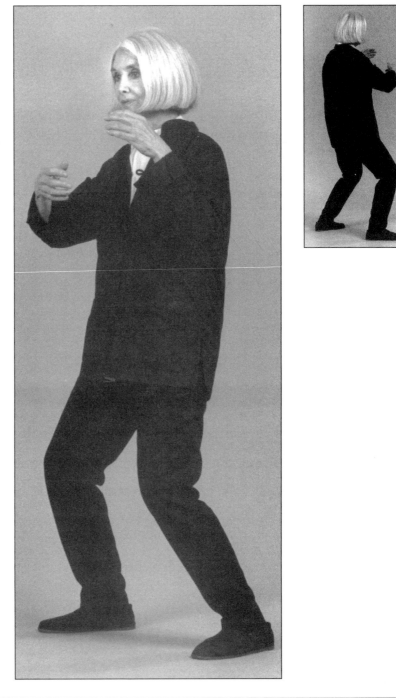

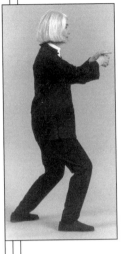

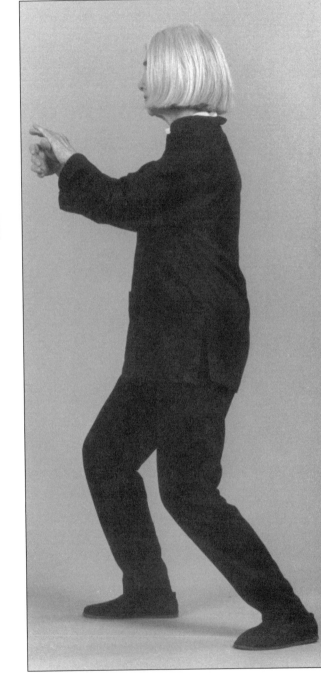

POSITION 3

You are now in the 70/30 Posture. The left hand has joined the right hand, left palm pressing lightly against the fatty part of the right thumb. Keep the left wrist and forearm in an unbroken line, gently curved. Sink your right hipbone and drop your left knee to feel even more relaxed and rooted in the stance.

POSTURE 7 — GRASP SPARROW'S TAIL, PUSH

POSITION 1

Continuing the flow, move 100 percent of your weight back into your left leg. As you shift, separate your hands and begin to drop your elbows, drawing the backs of the wrists toward the shoulders.

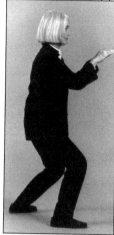

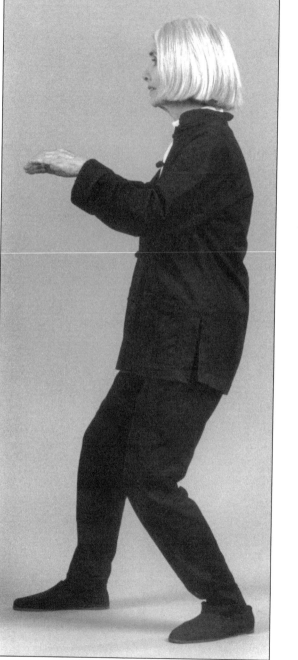

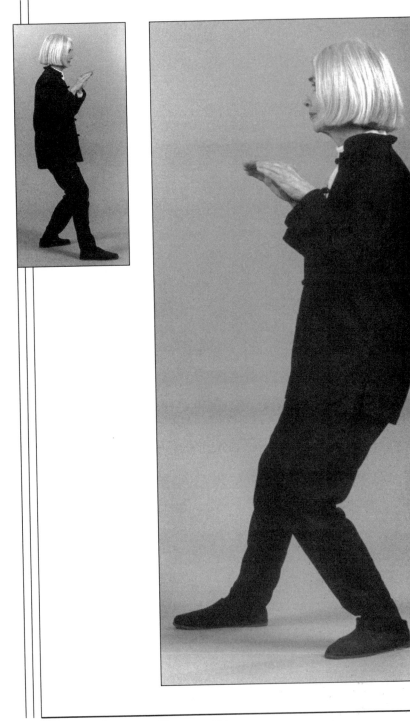

POSITION 2

Feel sand pour down from the wrists into the elbows as the arms move back. In this move and the next two, you will be shifting back and forth. Be sure not to bob your body up and down as you move, but keep on one even level, knees quarter-bent. Picture yourself moving through a low tunnel—you don't want to hit your head on the roof!

POSITION 3

Again moving forward, shift 70 percent of your weight back into your right leg. Your arms come with you and are parallel to each other (in profile they form a V shape) as they move forward for a push. The arms do not move by themselves. They are moved by the momentum of the shifting of the lower body.

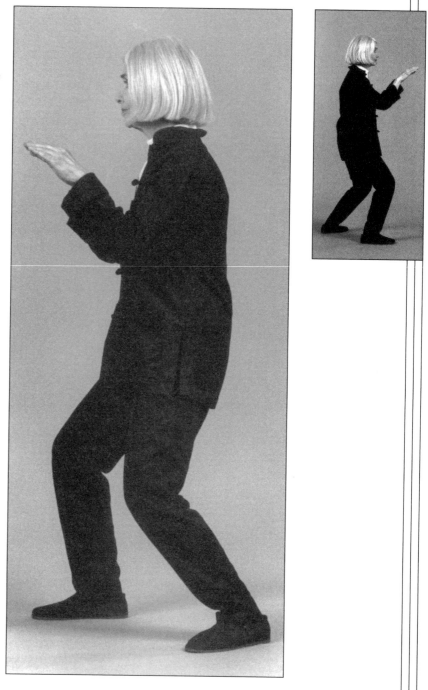

POSTURE 8 — SINGLE WHIP

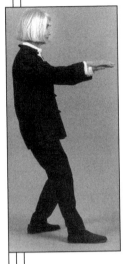

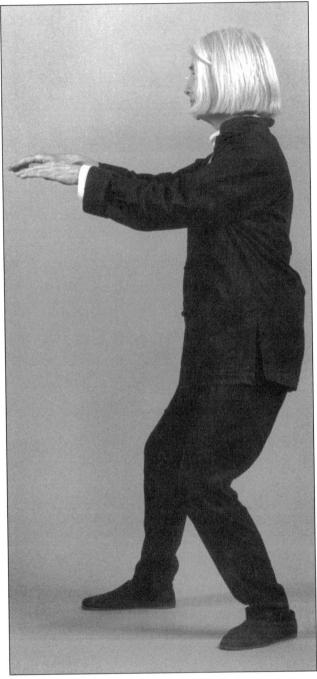

POSITION 1

Now again, all of your weight shifts back into your left leg. Leave your arms where they are and draw back from them so that as you move away, your arms stretch out and rest, as if floating on ocean water.

POSITION 2

You are sitting so far back on your left leg that the toes of your right foot come off the ground. Retain the perpendicular line from your head down through your spine—do not lean backward. You are loose and relaxed.

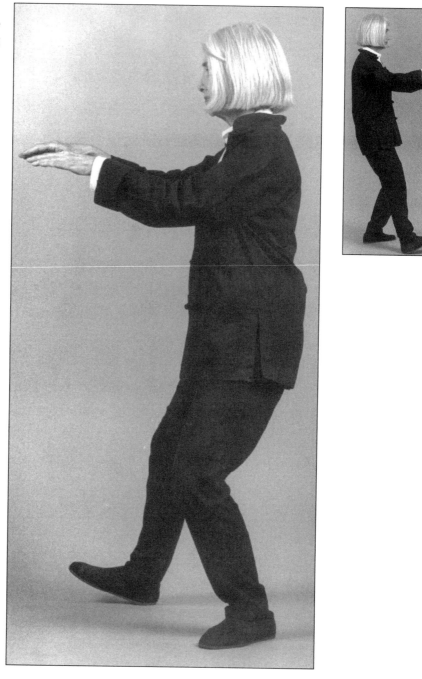

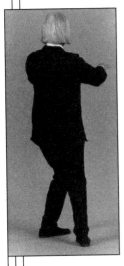

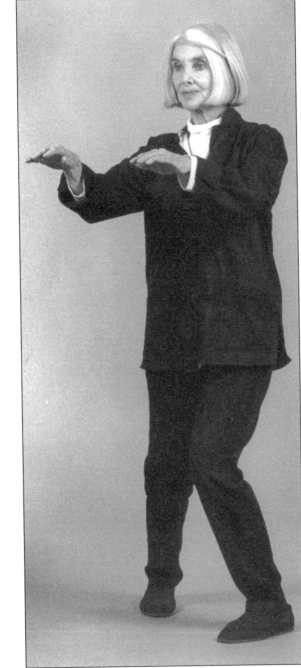

POSITION 3

Pivoting on the heel of your empty right foot, begin to turn your torso to the front (north), the right toes coming with you. Your arms are parallel to the ground. They do not move by themselves but are moved by the action of the turn, staying in line with the pelvic bones. Your right heel turns until the foot sets down flat, pointed straight ahead (north) and empty of weight.

POSITION 4

Keeping all your weight in your left leg, melt your left hipbone and continue revolving left as if turning on a carousel pole, toward the front left corner (northwest). The arms are never out of line with the pelvic bones. All the weight is still in the left leg; the right leg is hollow. Both knees are equally bent. This shape may be difficult to achieve at first; only turn as far as you can, keeping all of your weight in your left leg while maintaining a perpendicular balance.

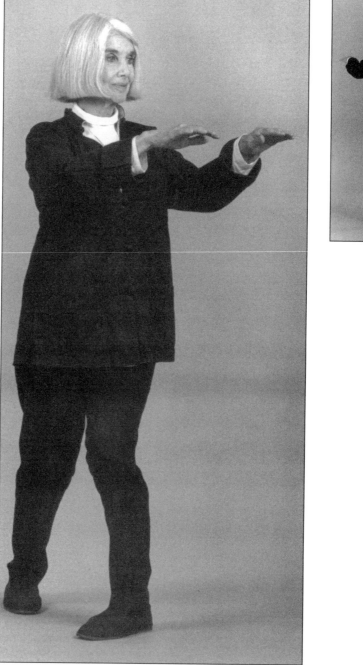

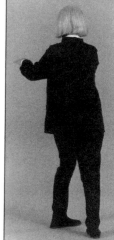

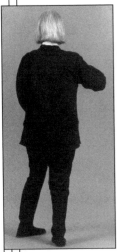

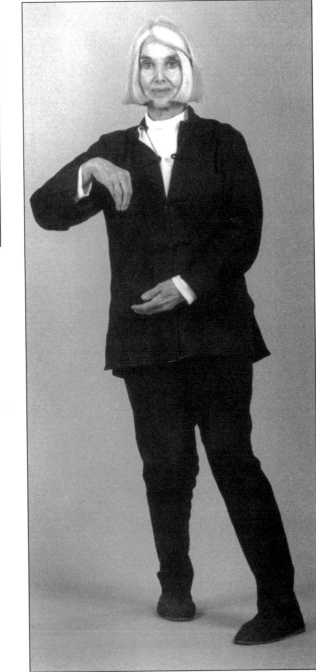

In the same slow rhythm, bring your entire body weight back on top of your right leg, filling that leg with sand as you completely empty your left leg, which becomes hollow. Simultaneously, your arms draw back toward your body. The right hand forms a bird's beak (the four fingers and thumb pinched together), just below your right armpit (see p. 13). The left hand positions itself by the right hip, in the shape of a plate to catch the imaginary crumbs that fall from the bird's beak. You are now in perfect plumb-line balance, from the top of your head, down your spine, through your tailbone, through the right leg, and into the center of the earth.

POSITION 6

Turn on the carousel pole to the right front corner (northeast). Pick up the heel of the empty left foot. Arms and hands remain as they are, right hand a bird's beak, left hand in the shape of a plate by the right hip.

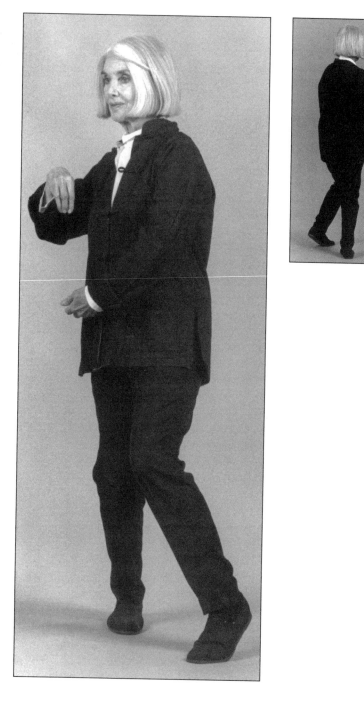

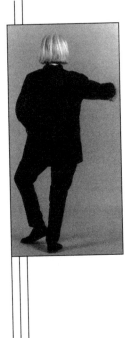

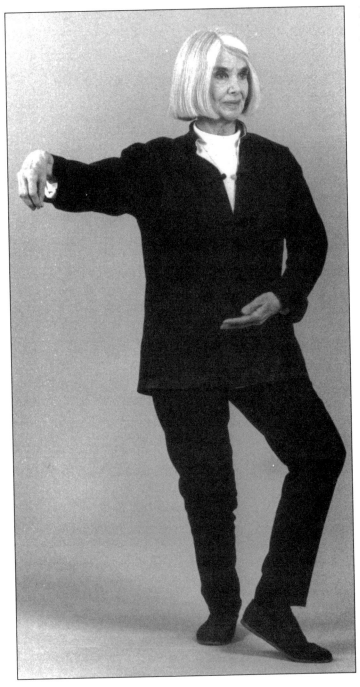

POSITION 7
Revolve your body on the carousel pole to the left as the heel of the left foot comes around to the right. Simultaneously, the bird's beak hand travels out at the same speed to the front right corner (northeast). These two actions must be done in unison.

POSITION 8

Leaving your bird's beak at the northeast corner, take a large low-to-the-ground step with your left foot (the heel touching first), and place the foot (empty) in the front left corner of the imaginary rectangle projected to the left wall (west). You are facing the front left corner (northwest). As you shift 70 percent of your weight into your left leg, your left palm slowly comes up the front of your body in an arc to your face. Again, the bird's beak arm stays where it is. Keep the elbow of the right arm slightly bent so there is no tension.

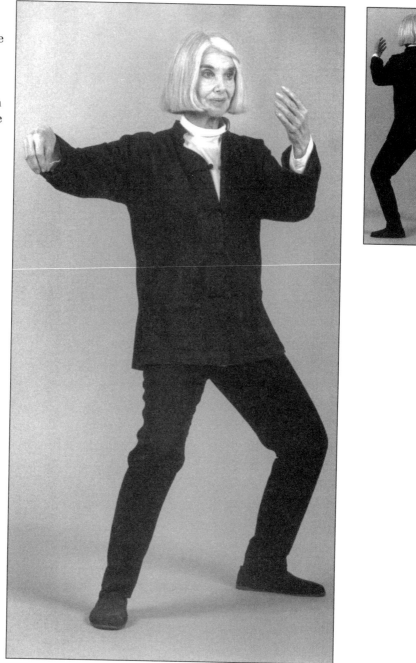

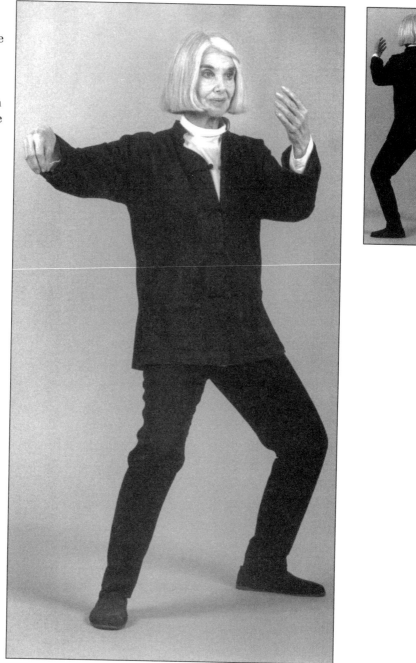

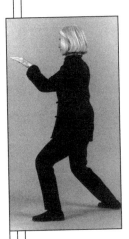

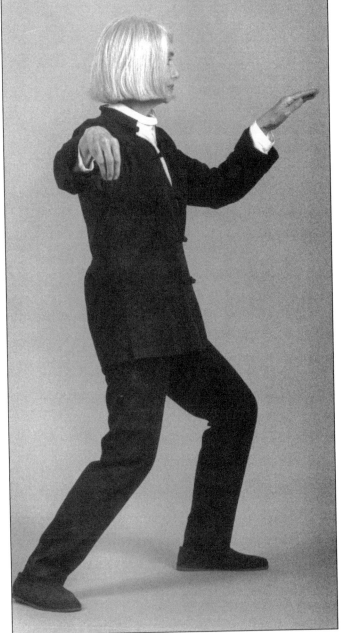

POSITION 9

At the last moment, as the toes of your right foot release, and you are pivoting on your right heel to turn directly to the left wall (west), the left palm turns over to face outward. You are now in the 70/30 Posture. Left hip drops; right knee drops. Your right hand is still in the shape of a bird's beak. Your left arm is directly in front of your left shoulder, the left hand in the shape of a swan's head (see p. 13).

POSTURE 9 — LIFT HANDS

POSITION 1

Letting the movement begin from the base of your spine, shift 100 percent of your weight into your left leg. The heel of the right foot peels off the ground. Let the right knee hang.

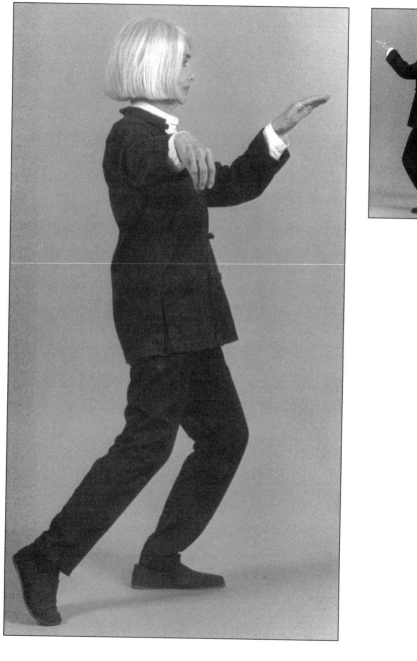

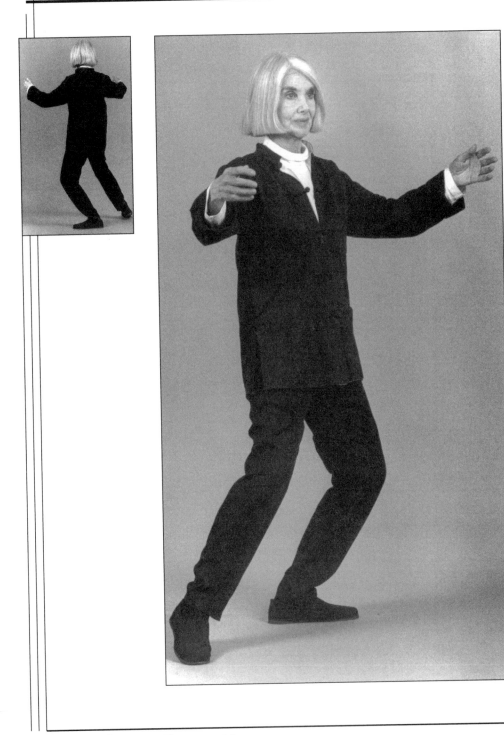

POSITION 2
Sink deeper down into your left leg as you turn your waist to the front left corner (northwest). Your right leg is empty, with just the toes touching the ground. Simultaneously, as you make the turn, open the palms of your hands to face each other, as if you are holding a very large beach ball.

Position 3

Turn your torso even more to the right to face almost front. Your bent (and empty) right leg releases and comes in front of your bent left leg, just the heel touching the ground. With the release of your right leg, your arms draw near each other in parallel lines, left palm facing right elbow. Both elbows are slightly bent, and the wrists bowed as if you are about to strum a harp. This is the only time the nose-over-navel rule is broken: Your body still faces the corner, but your head is now facing directly north.

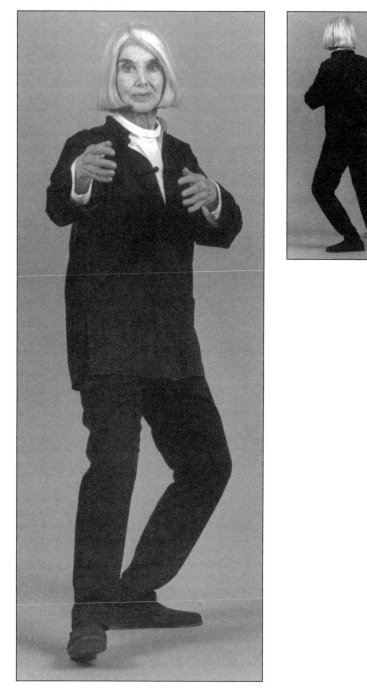

POSTURE 10 — LEAN FORWARD

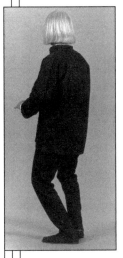

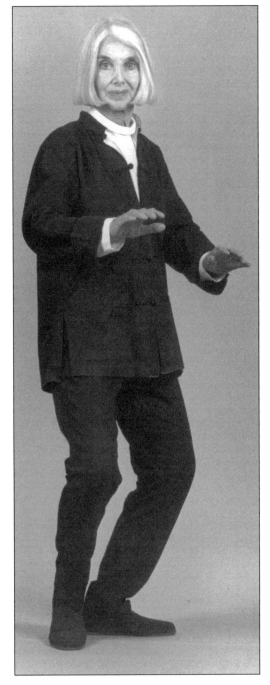

POSITION 1

With all of the weight still in your left leg, in the same slow rhythm bring the right foot back in front of the left foot, just the ball of the foot touching the ground. Leave the right foot empty of weight. Simultaneously, as the right foot comes back, the hands (heels of the palms leading) slowly descend, pushing down as if through the resistance of ocean water. Keep your chest deflated, tailbone dropped.

POSITION 2

The right palm is protecting your groin; the left hand is at your left side. The left leg has 100 percent of your weight. Keep the right leg hollow. Maintain your perpendicular balance (head to tailbone).

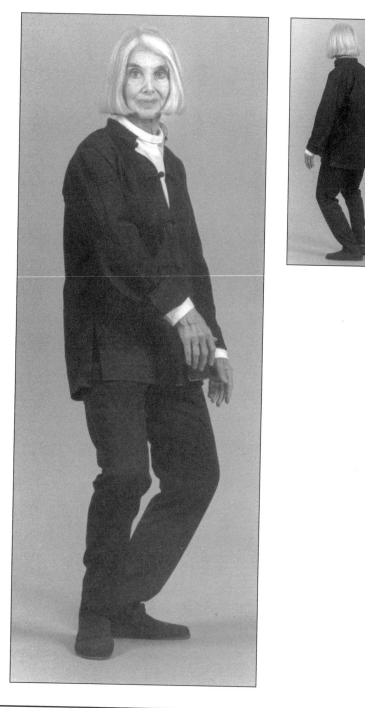

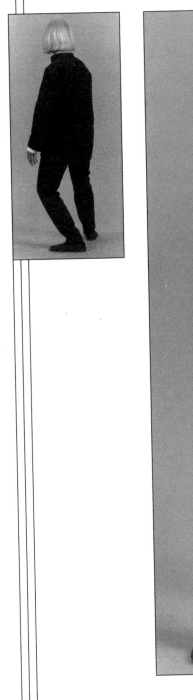

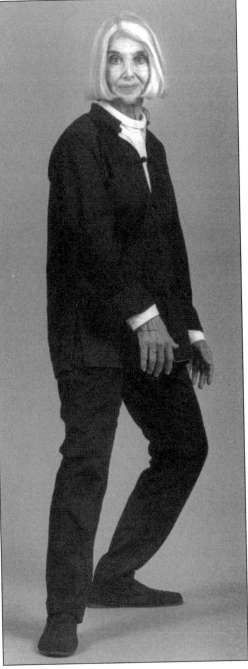

POSITION 3

Leaving all your weight in your left leg, sink even more weight into your left leg as you step forward again with your right foot, heel first, and place it down empty, toes facing north. Knees stay equally bent.

POSITION 4

Slowly move 70 percent of your weight into your right leg, your right arm still protecting the groin. At the same time, your left hand comes up, hiding behind the right arm, to rest between the elbow and the wrist, palm down. Don't punch your right elbow out, but keep the arm rounded, from the shoulder to the palm, like a bow.

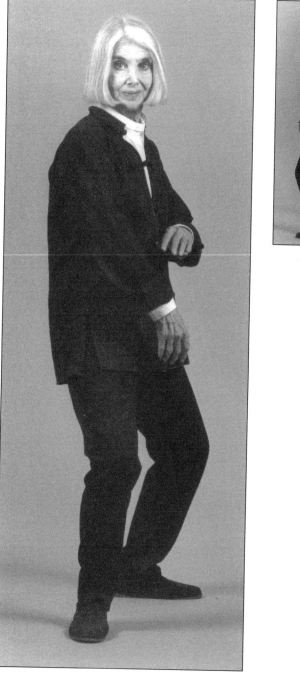

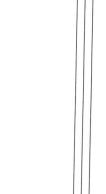

POSTURE 11 — STORK SPREADS ITS WINGS

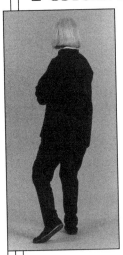

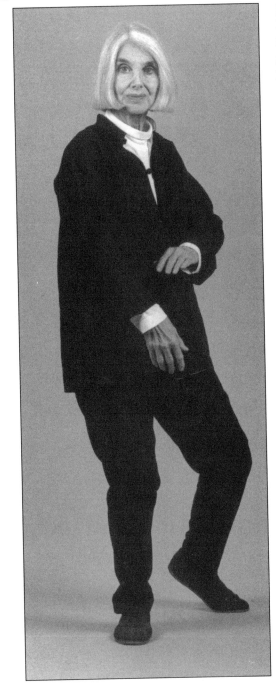

POSITION 1

From the base of the spine, move all of your weight into your right leg. The heel of your left foot releases. Your head is still facing straight ahead, your body toward the front left corner (northwest).

POSITION 2

Turn your waist to face directly to the left wall (west). Don't strain to square your hipbones; if you soften and drop your left hipbone as you turn, you will almost be facing directly west. The right leg will feel more rooted and balanced by this turn.

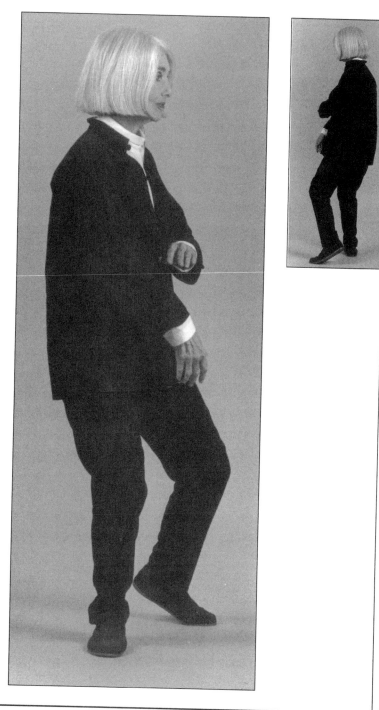

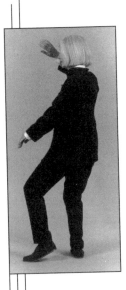

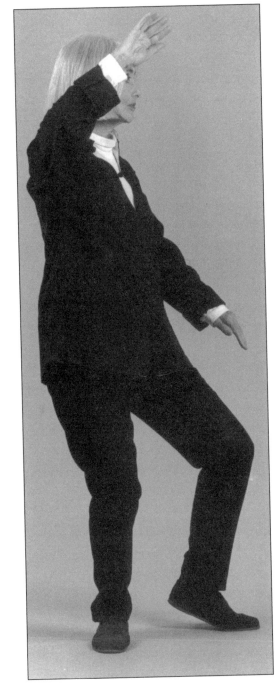

Position 3

Now release into a "spread of wings." The right hand comes up to protect your temple, palm facing out, as the left hand lowers to your side. Simultaneously, the empty left foot is released and comes in front of the right heel, just the toes touching, no weight in it. Your right "wing"—at the elbow—has risen to position itself at chin level. Try not to raise your shoulder as you bring your right arm up. Remember the resistance of the water pressure as you move your arms.

POSTURE 12 — BRUSH LEFT KNEE AND TWIST STEP

POSITION 1

Down floats the right arm from the temple, through the ocean water. As it slowly descends, keep the right elbow close to your body, and the palm will end up facing outward, at 6 on the clock. Your weight is still 100 percent in your right leg, and your hipbones are still facing directly toward the left wall (west).

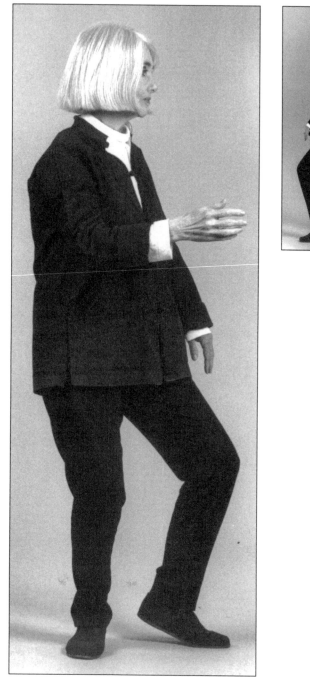

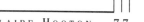

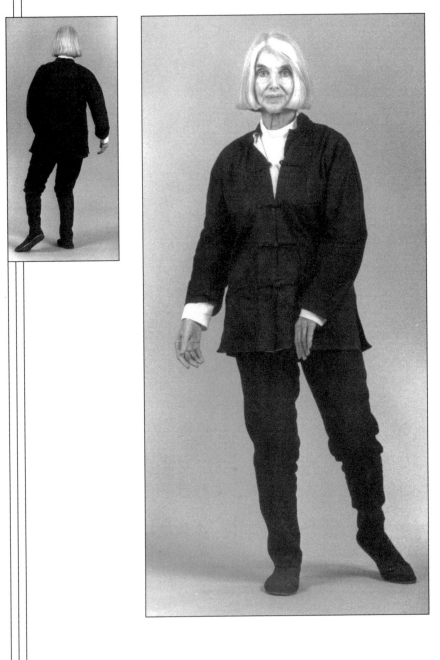

Position 2

By melting your right hipbone, turn your waist directly front (north). As you turn, bring your arms with you. Your right arm arrives at your side, and your left arm arrives between your thighs, with the left palm turned to face your left thigh. The left hand is positioned precisely—don't let it lose its energy as you prepare for the next move.

POSITION 3

Continuing the momentum, your right arm slowly rises to 9 on the clock. Imagine that the arm is being raised by a puppet string attached to the wrist. Keep your left hand placed exactly between your thighs, left palm facing your left thigh. Stay vertically balanced over your right leg.

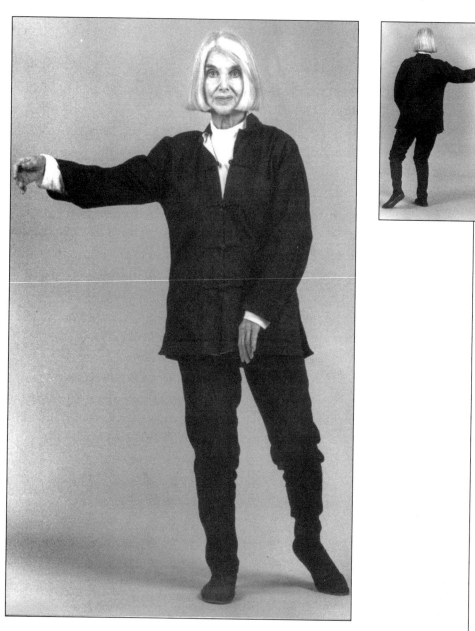

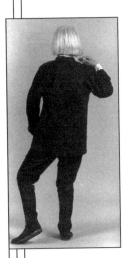

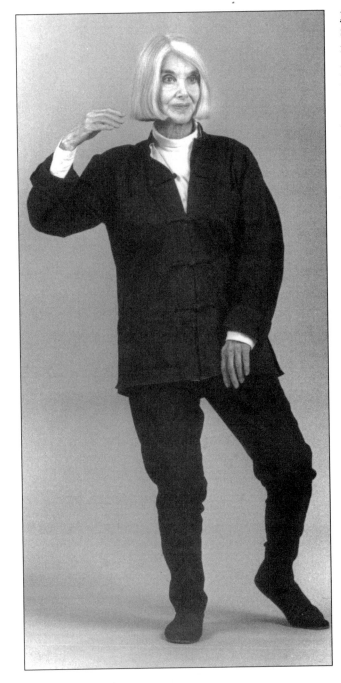

POSITION 4

Sink more weight into your right leg and melt your left hipbone to turn and face the front left corner (north-west). As you turn, drop your right elbow; your right palm comes with you and arrives just below your right earlobe. Elbow stays loose.

POSITION 5

Sink the weight into your right leg even more to root yourself and step out empty with your left leg, heel touching first, to the left corner of an imaginary rectangle projected directly toward the left wall (west). The left leg has no weight in it as you place it down. Keep the energy alive in your left hand by being conscious of the hand.

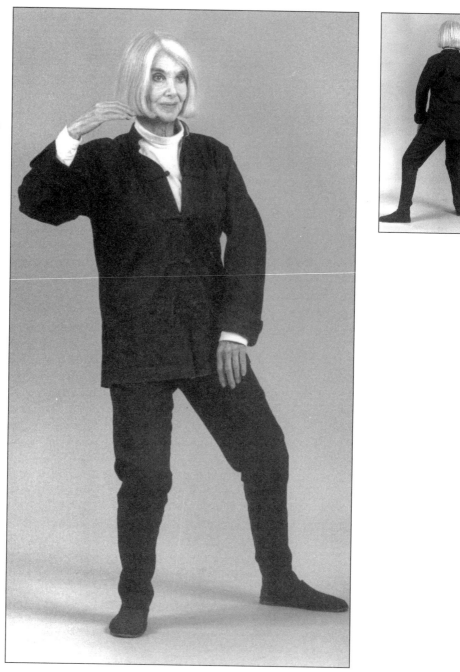

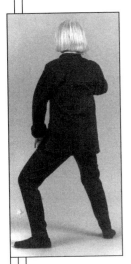

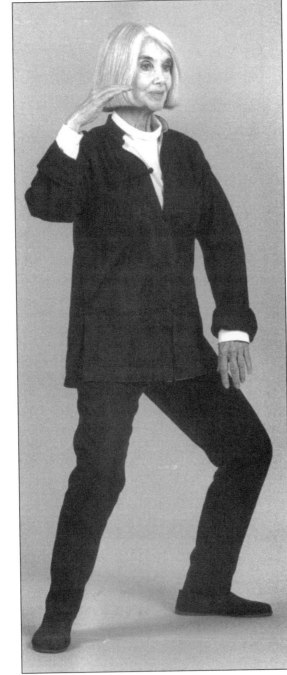

POSITION 6

You are facing the north-west corner of the room as you shift 70 percent of your weight into your left thigh without changing your hand positions.

POSITION 7

Continuing the momentum, release the toes of your right foot. As you pivot on the right heel, the action of the pelvis turning sends your left hand over the left knee, pushing the air. The left hand arrives at your left side. Simultaneously sink the right elbow so that the right palm comes forward directly in front of the right shoulder, into the Swan's Head position. You are now in the 70/30 Posture. Stay relaxed.

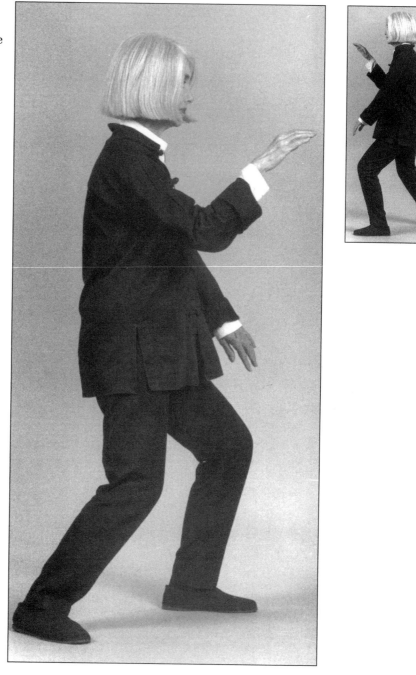

POSTURE 13 — PLAY THE GUITAR

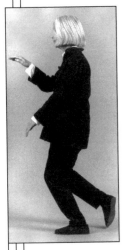

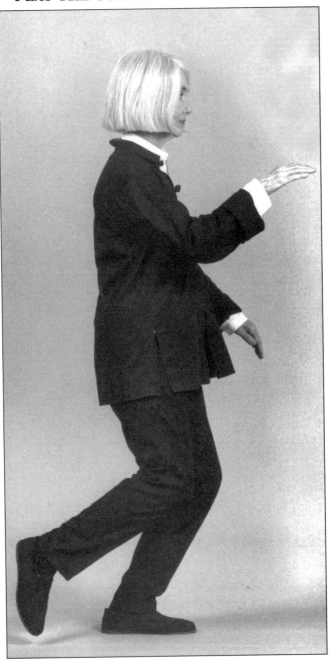

POSITION 1

Shift your weight completely into your left leg, leading with your tailbone, not your chest; your right foot is now off the ground. Balanced on your left foot, drop your right knee. Maintain a perpendicular line from the top of the head through the base of the foot and stay relaxed. Keep your right leg completely empty; do not point the toes.

POSITION 2

Still facing directly to the left wall (west), sink more weight into your left leg and step back with your right leg. Toes go down first, and the foot points directly front (north). All the weight is still in the left leg.

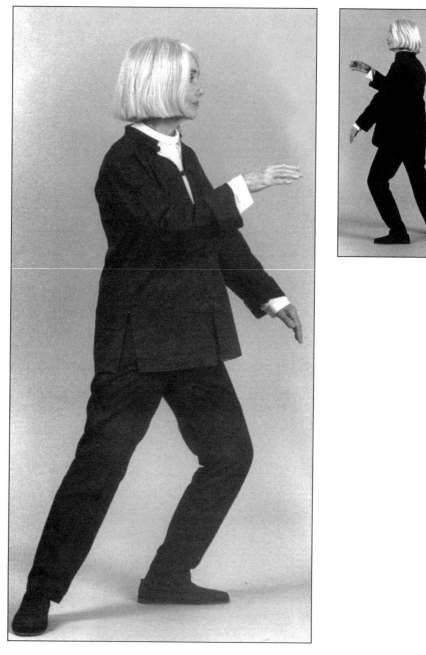

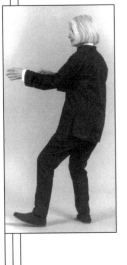

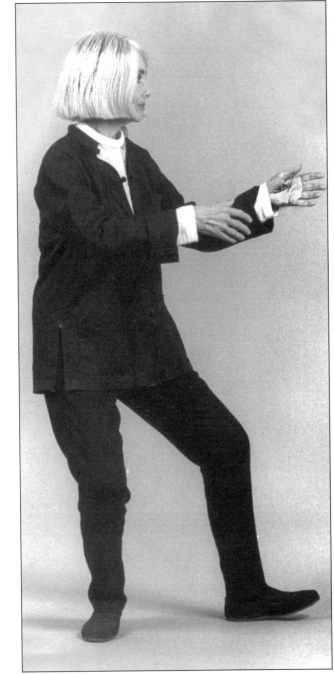

POSITION 3

Shift all the weight back into your right leg. As you do this, pick up the empty left leg and bring the left heel in front of the right heel, still with no weight in it. Simultaneously, the right arm draws back with the shift, right palm facing left elbow (the left arm is now further front than the right). Your arms assume the position of playing a guitar; both knees are equally bent.

POSTURE 14 — BRUSH LEFT KNEE AND TWIST STEP (REPEAT)

POSITION 1

Flop your left foot down and drop your arms as you turn your waist to the front (north). Your right arm is again at your side; your left arm is positioned between your thighs, palm facing your left thigh. Since the left palm holds the action of this step, don't let it become dead weight.

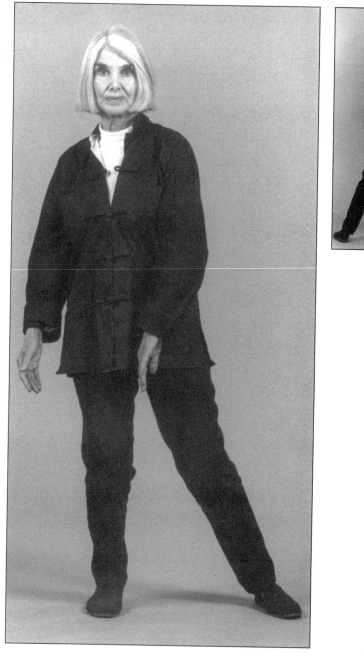

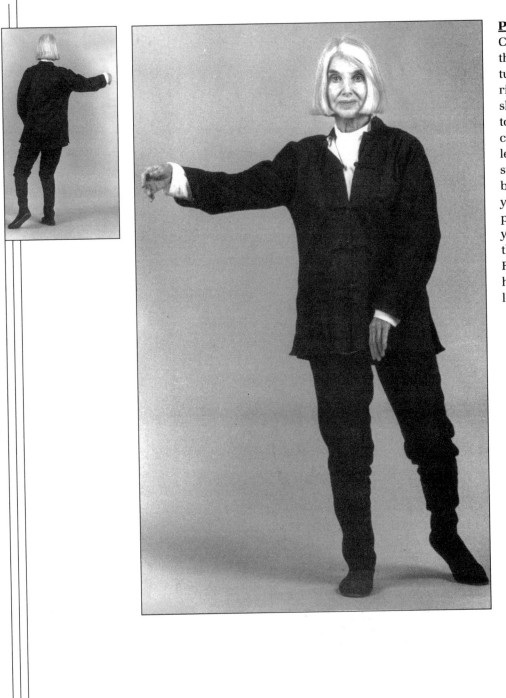

POSITION 2
Continuing the momentum, your right arm slowly rises to 9 on the clock. Your left hand stays between your thighs, palm facing your left thigh. Release the heel of the left foot.

POSITION 3

Turn and face the front left corner (northwest). As you turn, your right elbow drops down, and your right palm comes with you and arrives just below your right earlobe.

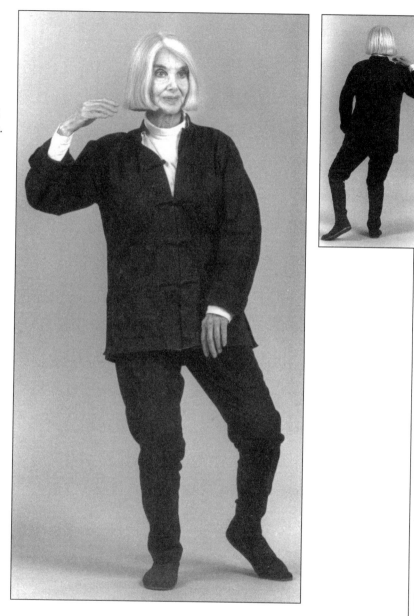

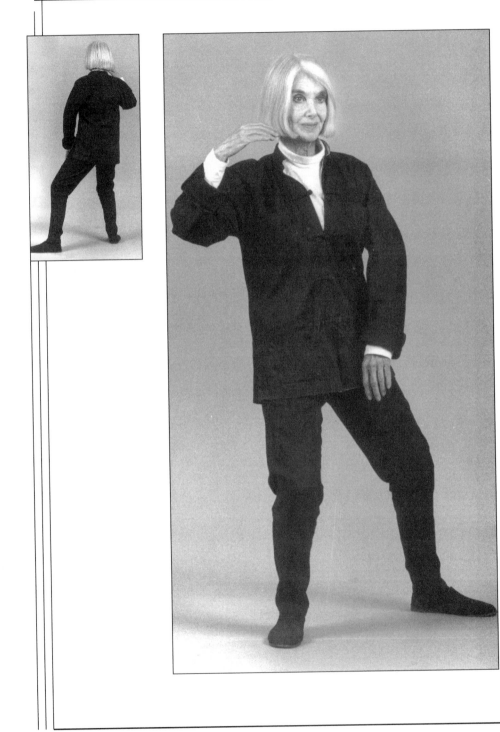

POSITION 4

Sink more weight into your right leg and step out with your left leg, heel touching first, into a rectangle projected directly toward the left wall (west). Be sure to step far enough to the left so that your legs will be shoulder distance apart—no weight is in the left leg as you set it down. Your left hand is between your thighs, right palm under right earlobe.

POSITION 5

Still facing the corner, shift 70 percent of your weight into your left leg. As you release your right toes (unhinge the gate), pivot on the heel and turn directly to the left wall (west). From the force of the turn, your left hand again brushes across your knee without touching it.

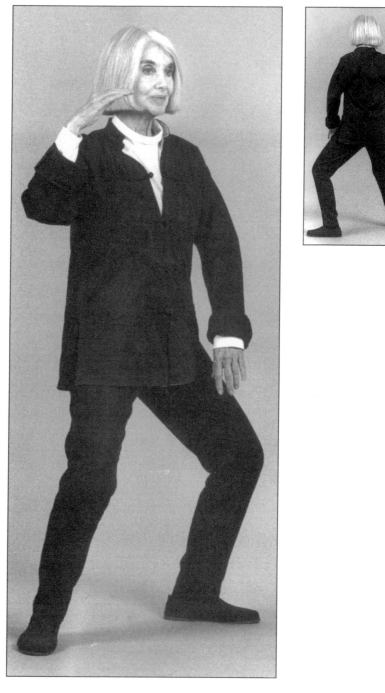

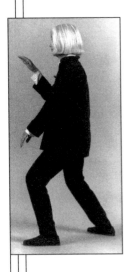

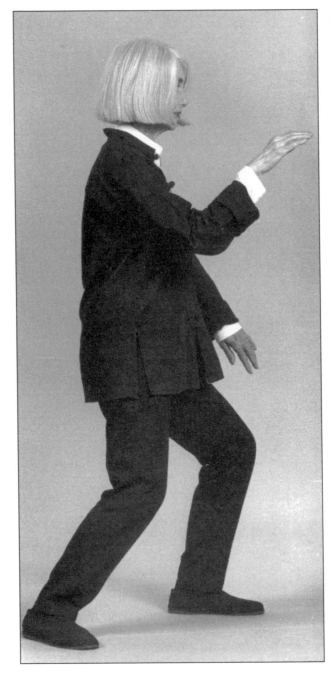

POSITION 6
The left hand arrives at your left side. At the same time, your right elbow drops with the turn of the waist, and the right hand flows forward into the Swan's Head position.

POSTURE 15—STEP FORWARD, DEFLECT DOWNWARD, PARRY & PUNCH

POSITION 1

With all of your weight, carry your whole upper body back onto your right leg, release the toes of your left foot, and turn your waist to the back corner (southwest). As you shift and turn, your arms descend and surround your left thigh, palms facing your body.

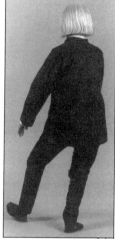

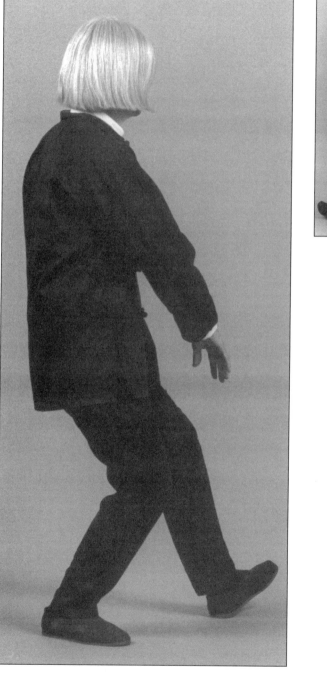

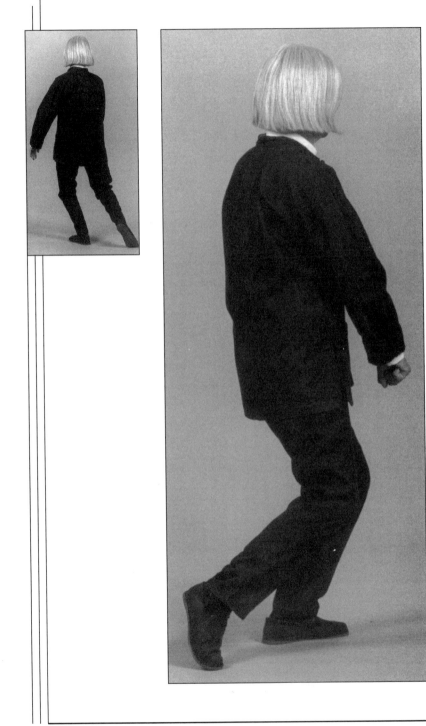

POSITION 2

Pushing your tailbone forward, slowly shift 100 percent of your weight into your left leg. As you're moving, the heel of the right foot peels off the ground. Simultaneously make a fist with your right hand. Keep your chest deflated, tailbone down.

POSITION 3

Make sure your hipbones are still facing the back corner as you place your empty right foot at a right angle to the arch of the left foot—far enough from the left foot that you will be able to bend your knees in order to drop your torso.

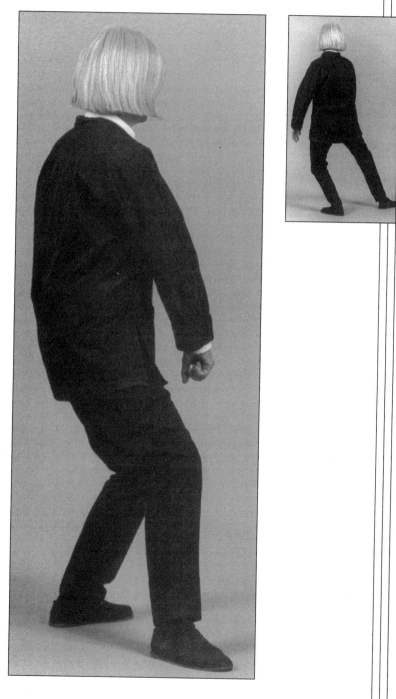

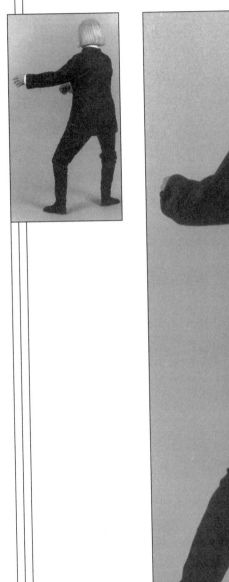

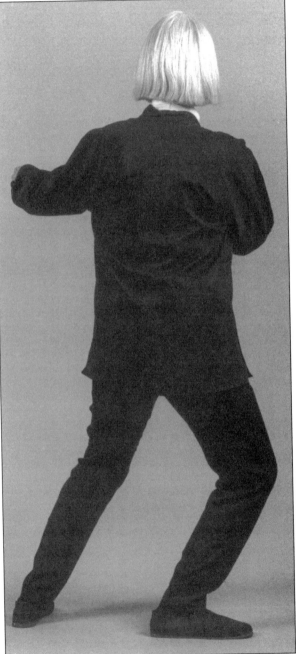

POSITION 4

Still facing the corner, begin to shift most of your weight into your right leg as your arms, in unison, come up at your left side. The right fist arrives at the left side of your chest, and the left arm stretches out at your left side, as if your two arms are about to haul in a net of fish. Keep your knees bent.

POSITION 5

Release the heel of your left foot. Turn right as you circle your waist to the front left corner (northwest). Bend and sink your right elbow near your chest during the turn so that your right fist comes close to your chin. The left palm has circled with the move and is now protecting the left side of your face.

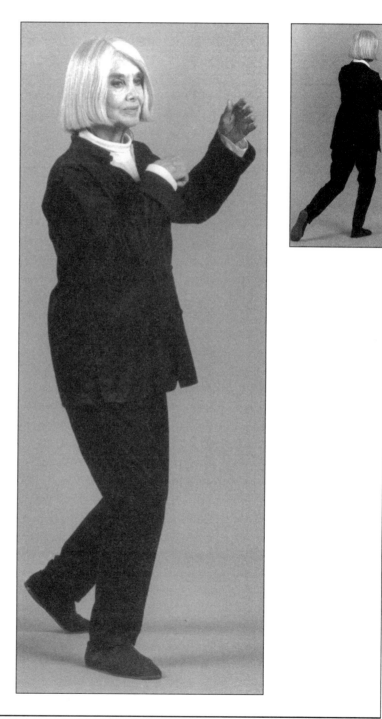

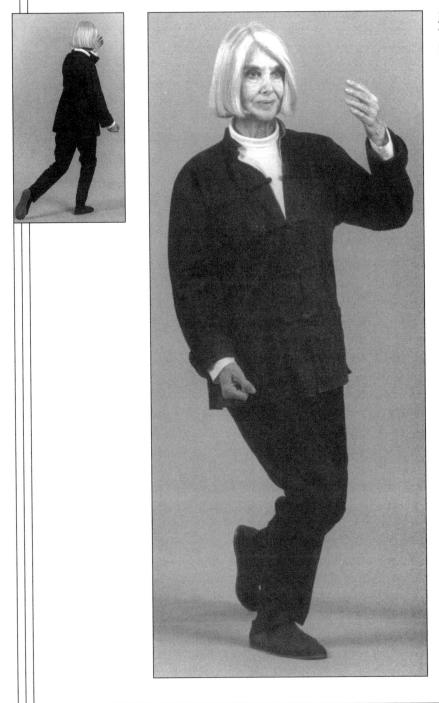

POSITION 6

Turn your waist even more to the right as you drop your fist by your side. Do not lean to the right as you release your right arm. Maintain your perpendicular balance. There is no weight in the left leg.

POSITION 7

Sink more weight into your right leg and step forward and to the left with your empty left leg. Place the foot, heel first, directly facing the wall (west) and into the front left corner of the rectangle. Be sure to place the left foot far enough to the left so that the feet are shoulder distance apart.

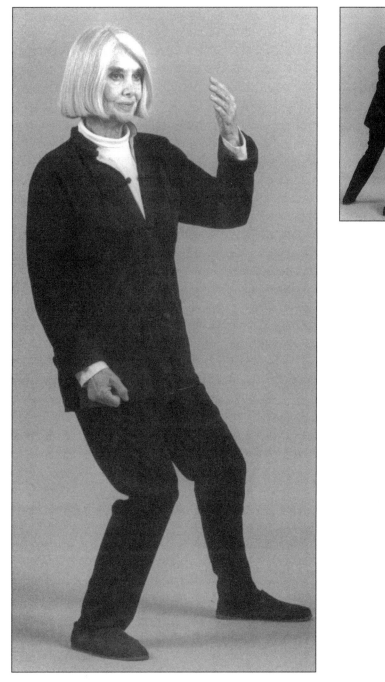

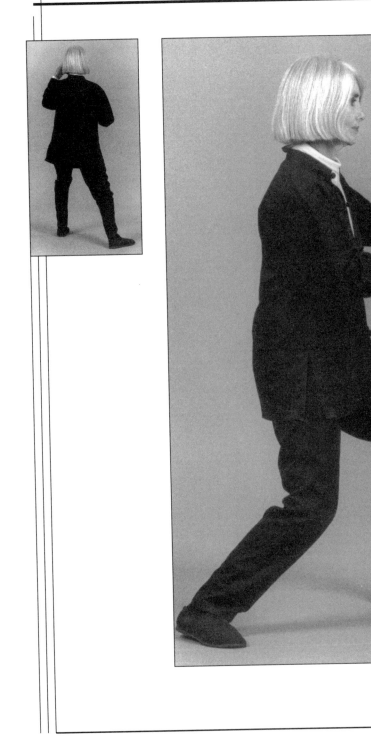

POSITION 8

Shift 70 percent of your weight into your front left leg as your right forearm ascends, as if lifted by a puppet string attached to the wrist; the hand is still a fist. Your right elbow bends into a right angle, at waist level. Your left palm is still protecting your head.

POSITION 9

Relax your left hip and sink down more in the 70/30 Posture as your left hand comes down to your side and your right fist, in unison, moves straight out in front of you into the "punch."

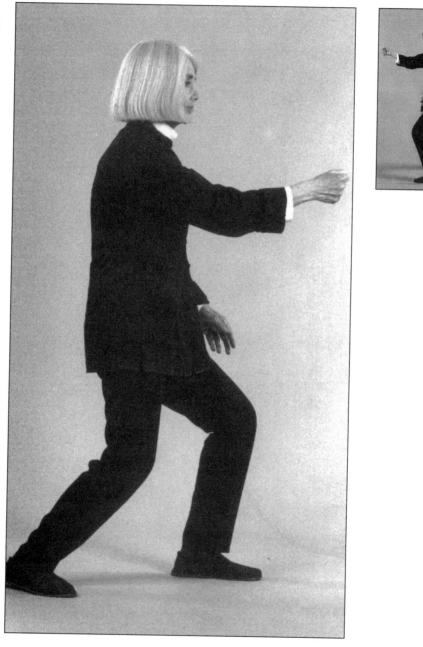

POSTURE 16 — GET THE NEEDLE AT THE SEA BOTTOM

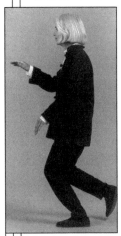

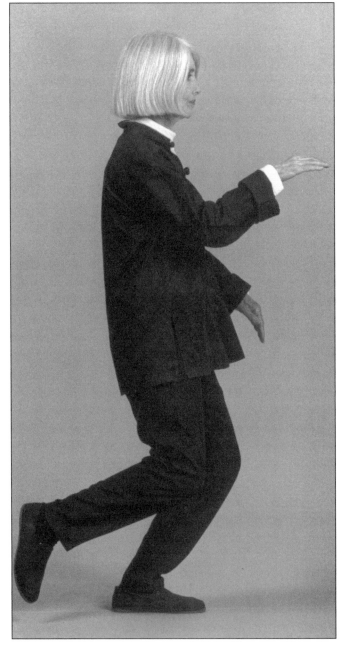

POSITION 1
Open up your fingers and stand on your left leg. Your right foot comes off the ground. Maintain your perpendicular balance, chest deflated, tailbone down, head as if suspended by a string from above.

POSITION 2

Sink a little more weight into your left leg to step back with your right foot (toes go down first) and place it just where it was before, at a 45-degree angle, with no weight in it.

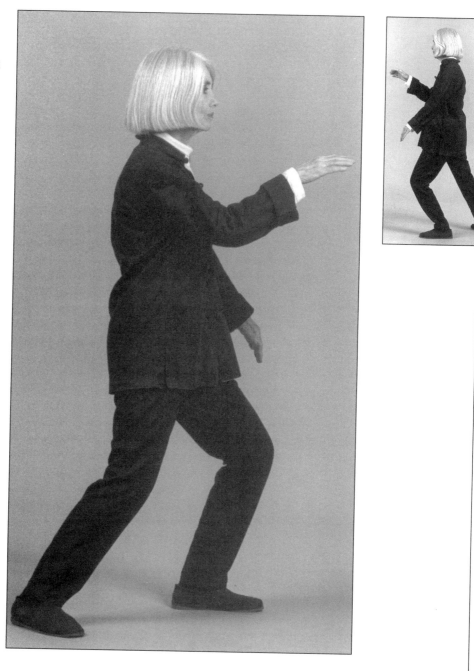

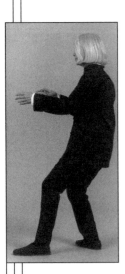

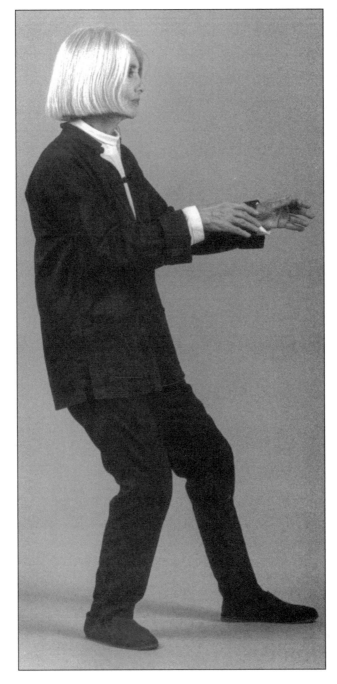

POSITION 3
As you slowly shift 100 percent of your weight into your right leg, your right hand moves back with you, drawing closer to your body; in unison, your left hand rises, because of the weight sinking into the right leg.

POSITION 4

The heel of your empty left foot releases, and the left foot moves over in front of the right heel, just the ball of the foot touching the ground. In unison, place the fingers of your left hand on top of the tendon of your right index finger. The fingers of the right hand are loose and begin to aim toward the ground. All tiny moves are done with the same rhythm as the large ones—without any jerking or abruptness.

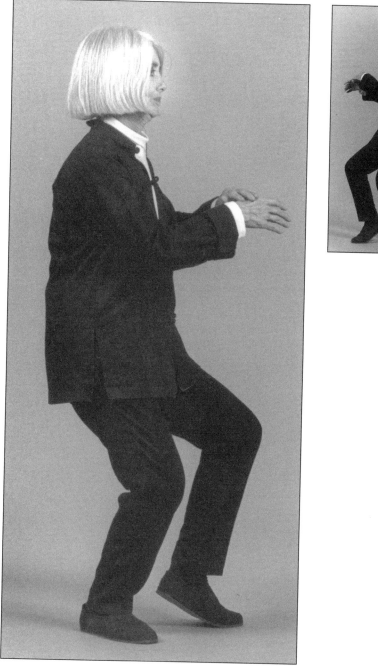

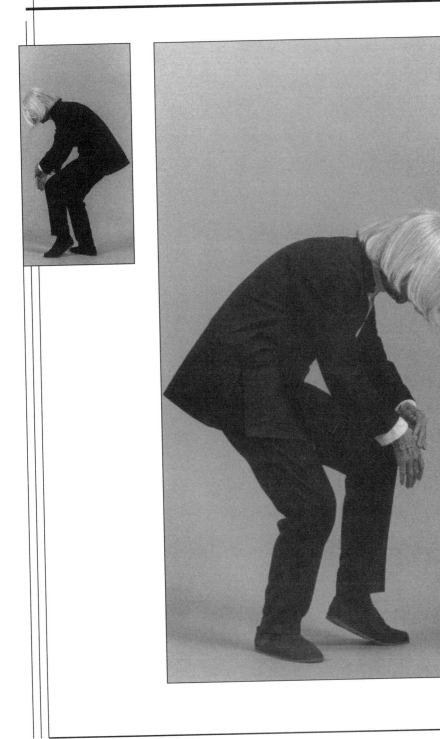

POSITION 5

With your tailbone
under you, and
your right fingers
aimed at the
ground, fold your
body over as you
slowly descend.

POSITION 6

Continuing down, keep your tailbone under you as you curve into an egg shape. Don't lean at all on your left leg; all the weight is in your right leg as you descend. Keep the same slow rhythm throughout the drop until your fingertips arrive close to the ground. Make sure you are facing directly toward the left wall (west) and your arms are centered between your legs.

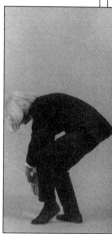

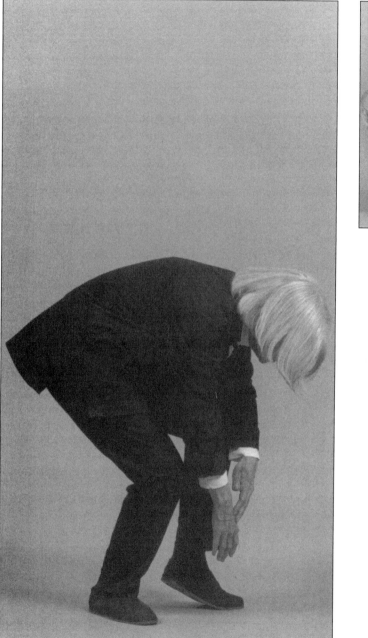

Posture 17 — Spread Arm Like a Fan

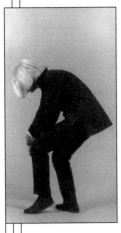

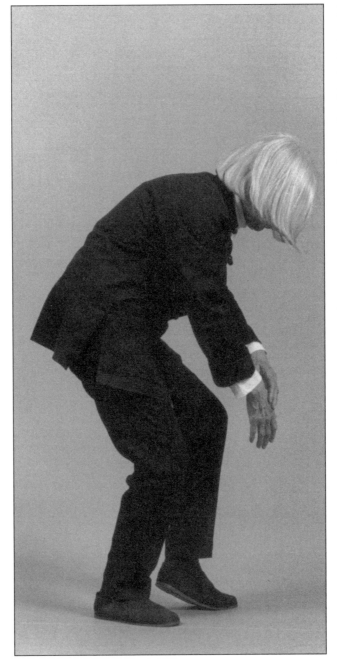

Position 1

In the same slow rhythm, and keeping your tailbone under you, bring your body up again until you are vertical. There is still no weight in your left leg.

POSITION 2

Once you are vertical, sink more weight into your right leg and you will feel as if you've turned a bit to the right. The fingers of your left hand are still resting on top of the tendon of your right index finger.

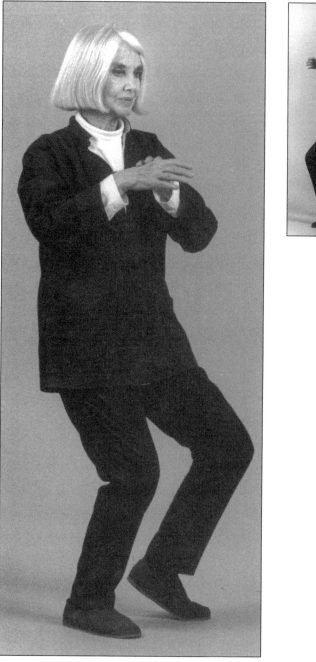

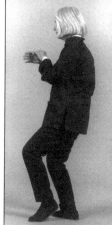

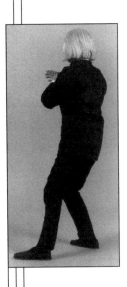

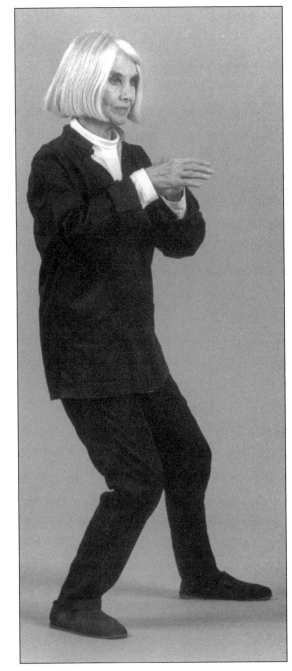

POSITION 3
Step out with your left leg, heel first, into the left front corner of an imaginary rectangle, toes projected directly toward the left wall (west). Be sure you establish shoulder distance between your feet.

POSITION 4

As you shift 70 percent of your weight into your left leg, turn your body a little to the left, which will bring your arms in over your left thigh. Your entire torso is now squared directly to the left wall (west).

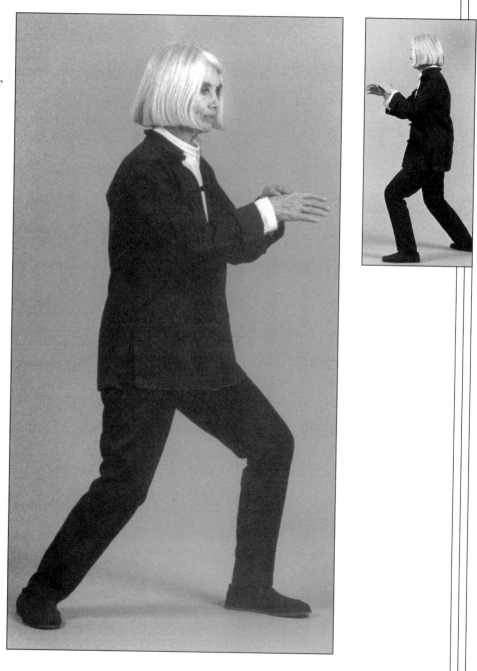

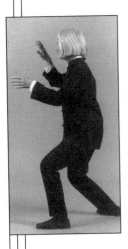

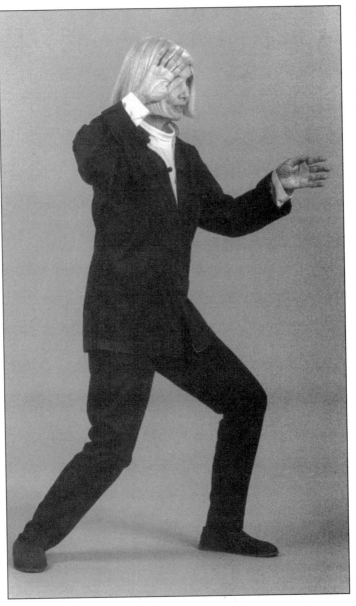

POSITION 5
At the last moment, turn your body slightly to the right while your arms spread out into the shape of a fan: the back of the right palm comes up to protect your temple while the left arm slices down into a right angle, stopping at tabletop level.

POSTURE 18—TURN AND STRIKE WITH BACK FIST, CHOP WITH FINGERS

POSITION 1

Shift 100 percent of your weight into your right leg. Your left forearm comes back with you. Your right palm stays at your temple. The toes of your left foot release, moving you even further back onto your right leg.

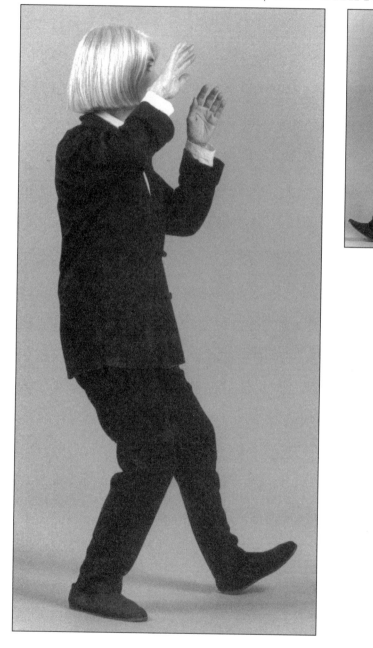

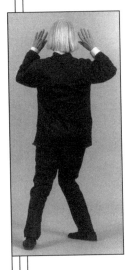

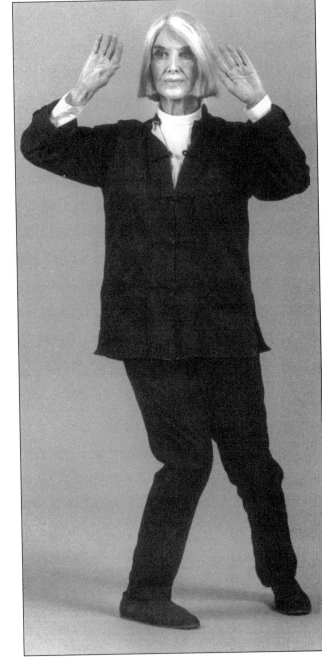

POSITION 2

Pivoting on the left heel, soften your right hip and turn your waist directly front (north). The toes of your left foot come with you and point straight ahead to the front (north). As you turn, the back of the left hand turns over so that now the backs of both hands protect your temples. All of your weight is still in your right leg. Your left leg is empty. Be sure your right hipbone does not push out but stays directly over the right leg.

POSITION 3

Imagine pouring all of the sand into your left leg. As you shift, your arms move down to protect your body, left palm facing your chest, right palm facing your groin. All movements are slow and steady. Keep the flow continuous.

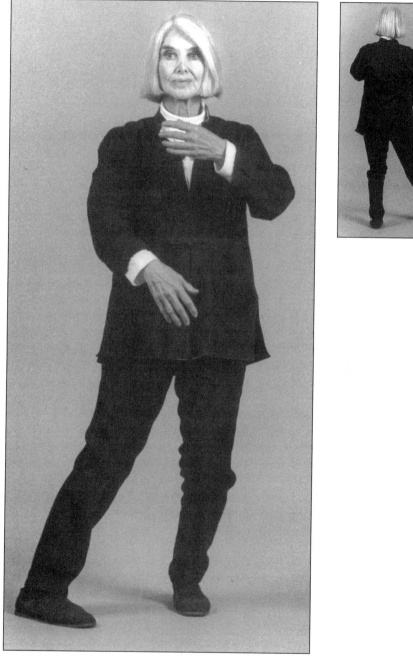

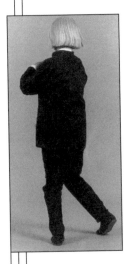

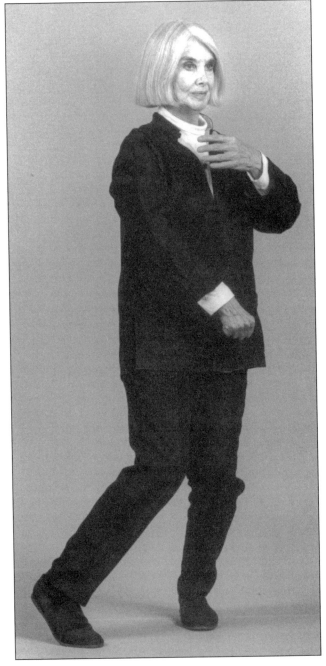

POSITION 4

Melt to the left, which will sink more weight into the left leg. As you turn to the left, the heel of your right foot releases and your right hand shapes into a fist. Keep your head up, as if suspended by a string.

POSITION 5

Sink more weight into your left leg, turning your body to the right, as if drilling a hole circularly into the earth. Your empty right leg pivots on the ball of the foot as you're turning, and the right heel comes around to the left. At the same time, by dropping your right elbow and keeping it close to your chest as you turn, the right fist swings up near your right shoulder.

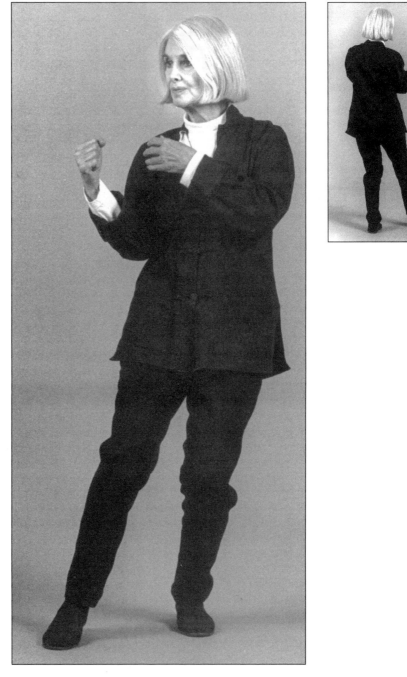

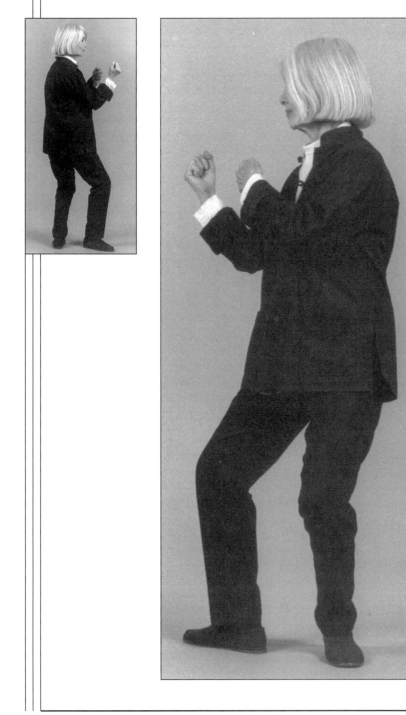

POSITION 6

Sink even more weight into the left leg as you raise your right foot slightly off the ground and set it down again, at the same even speed, at a 45-degree angle, projected directly toward the right wall (east). It touches the ground without any weight in it.

POSITION 7

Move all of your weight into your right leg. As you shift, your right hand, still a fist, pulls backward, knuckles down—as if stretching an elastic band. Your left hand extends forward in front of the right thigh, palm facing down. Simultaneously release your left leg and place it empty, heel first, in the left front corner of an imaginary rectangle projected directly toward the right wall (east).

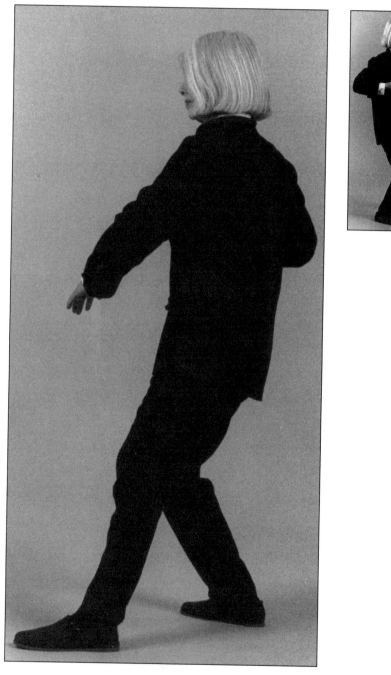

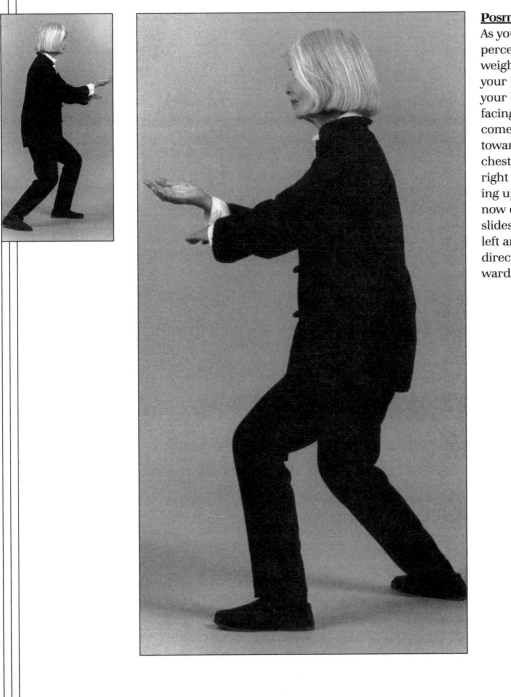

POSITION 8

As you move 70 percent of your weight into your left leg, your left palm, facing down, comes back toward your chest, and your right palm, facing up, fingers now extended, slides over the left and extends directly forward (east).

POSTURE 19 — WITHDRAW AND PUSH

POSITION 1

Turn your waist to the left as your right arm continues around in a circle, until the right elbow is in front of the left wrist. Be sure not to turn your shoulders; the move is initiated solely by the turn of the lower abdomen.

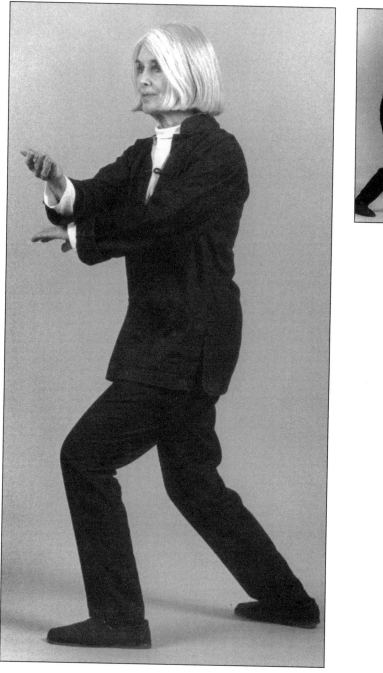

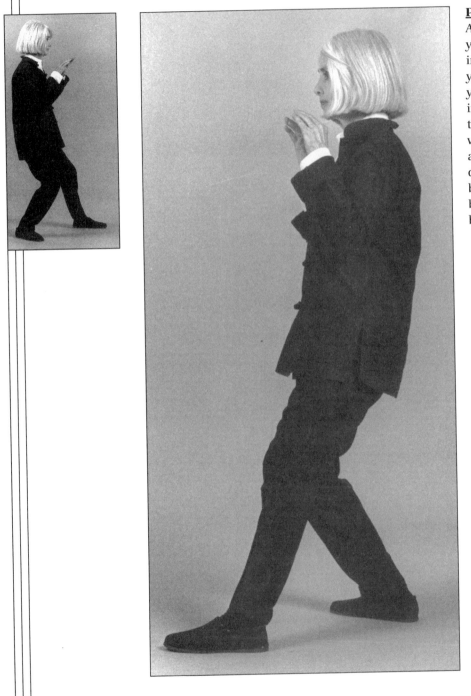

POSITION 2

As you shift all your weight back into your right leg, your elbows drop, your hands cross in front of you, and the backs of the wrists turn and arrive at the shoulders. Left leg becomes hollow; both knees are bent.

POSITION 3

Leaving your arms where they are, in the same slow rhythm bring your empty left foot slowly back and place it at a 45-degree angle under your left shoulder.

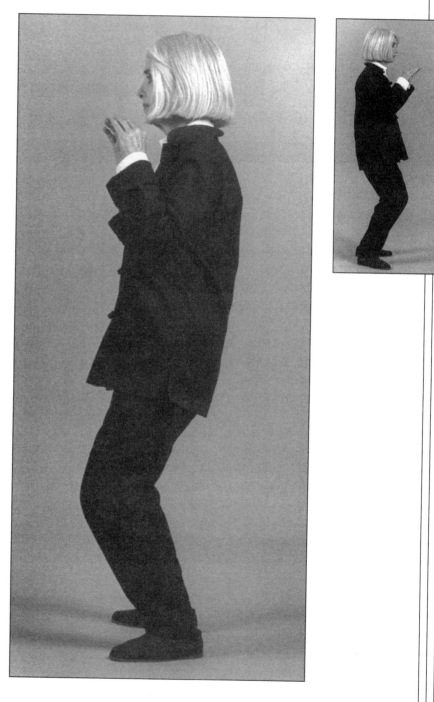

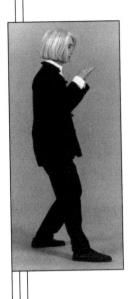

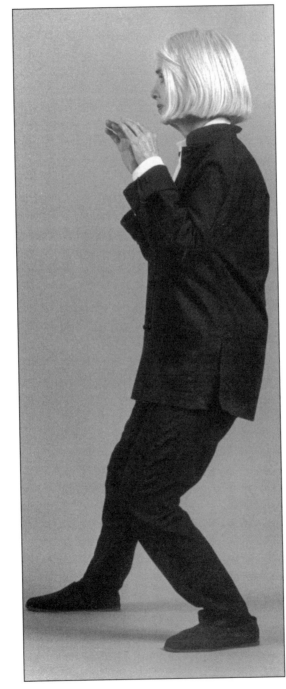

POSITION 4
In the same slow rhythm—
do not change your
speed—place your empty
right leg in the right front
corner of an imaginary
rectangle projected directly
toward the right wall (east).

POSITION 5

Now, with your tailbone (not your chest) leading, shift into the 70/30 Posture. As you shift 70 percent of your weight into your right leg, your arms move forward and away from your shoulders but no further than the momentum of the move carries them. The profile of the arms looks like a V. To be relaxed in this shape, soften your right hip and drop your left knee.

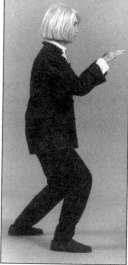

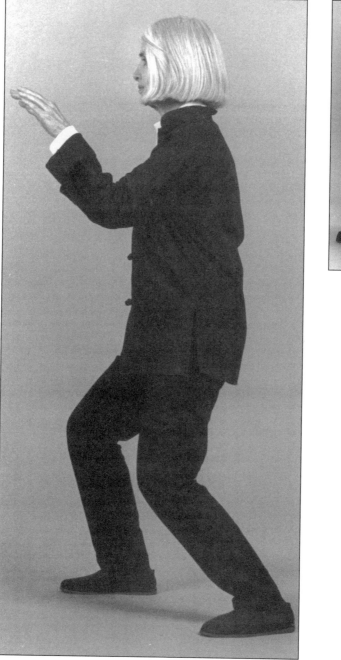

POSTURE 20 — CROSSING HANDS, PRELIMINARY CLOSURE

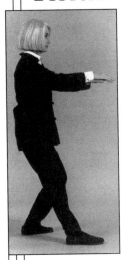

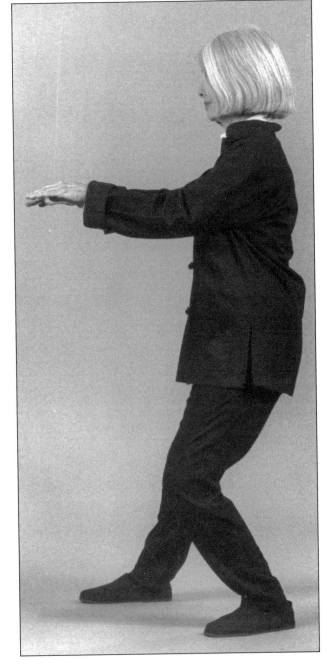

POSITION 1
Leave your arms in front of you and sit back away from them, moving your upper body, as one piece, onto your left leg. Do not lean backward as you move back. Your arms rest as if on ocean water. Feel the buoyancy of the water. Be very aware that your head is suspended by a string from above.

POSITION 2

Let go of your right hip completely. The toes of your right foot come off the ground. Keep your chest deflated, your tailbone down, and your rib cage directly on top of your pelvis.

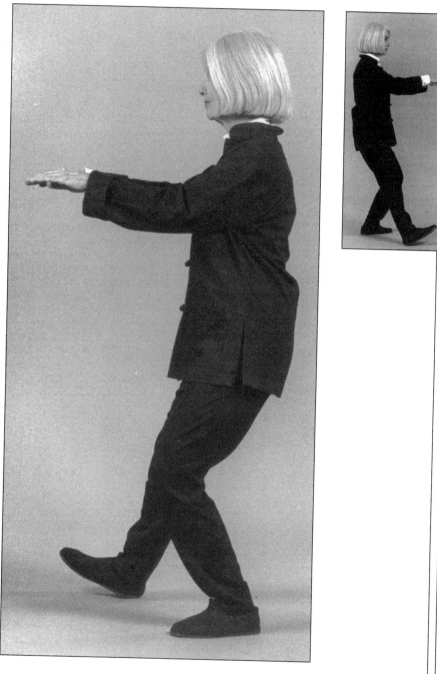

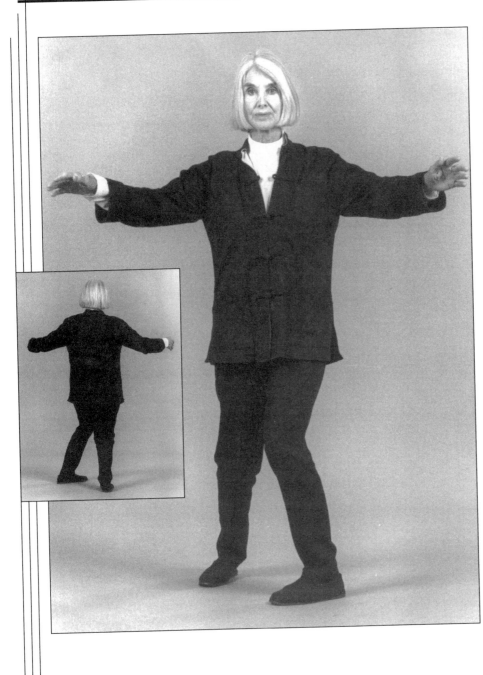

POSITION 3

Pivoting on the right heel, melt your left hipbone and slowly turn to the front (north), leaving your right arm where it is. With your left arm, moved by the momentum of the turn, describe a large arc across the front of your body. The right toes arrive directly front (north) just as the left arm arrives stretched out at your left side. Your pelvic bones are now directly front (north). Your left leg has not moved and is still carrying all the weight.

POSITION 4

Shift 100 percent of your weight into your right leg. Your relaxed arms slowly descend in unison with the rooting of the right leg. Simultaneously, the heel of your left foot releases, and you pivot on the ball of the foot so that it straightens to face front (north).

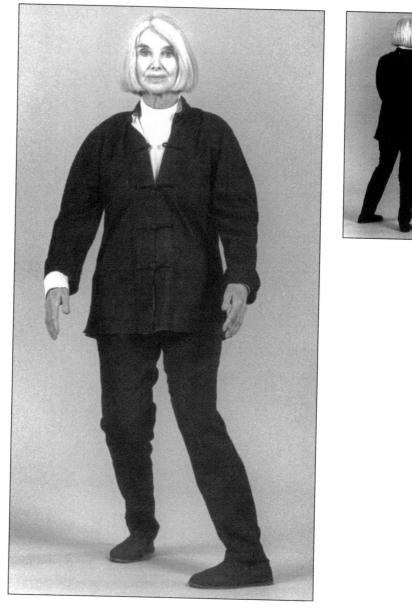

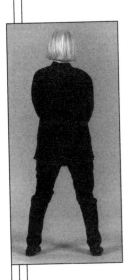

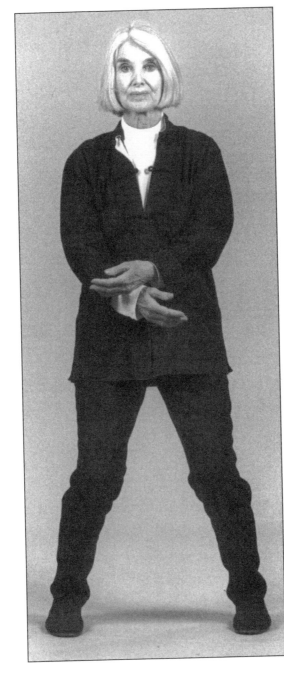

POSITION 5

Sink more into the ground with your right leg. Step back with your empty left foot and place it under your left shoulder, parallel with the right foot. With the knees bent, sink your weight evenly into both thighs as the right wrist crosses under the left wrist.

POSITION 6

Sinking more weight into both legs, your arms slowly rise to the front of your chest. Keep a nice open space—in the shape of a beach ball—between your chest and arms.

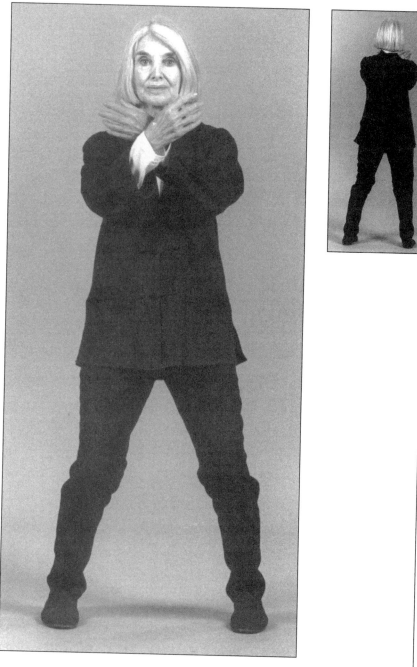

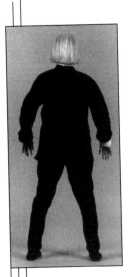

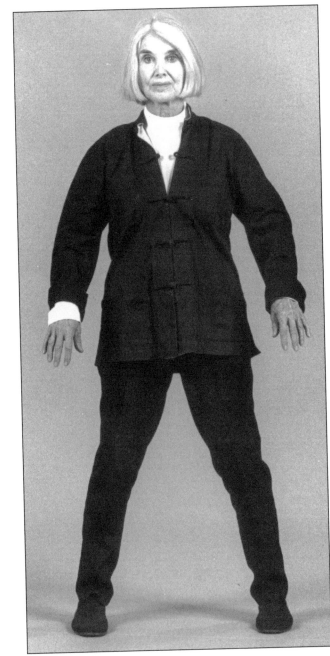

POSITION 7

Let the string attached to the crown of your head pull your body slowly upward as the arms slowly descend, as if pushing down through ocean water, and return to your sides with the backs of the wrists facing the front (north).

You have now completed the first third of the Yang-style Short Form.

THE TWELVE MOST COMMON MISTAKES

It is my experience as a teacher over the years that students really don't know how their bodies look as they're performing the steps. They have no idea they may be leaning forward or backward, veering to the right or left. They don't realize that a hip could be pushed out of place or their shoulders might be raised up. The following mistakes are chosen because they are so frequently made. By alerting you to these common errors, you will become aware of how easy it is to slip into incorrect postures. You will then be able to watch that you carry out your body direction with accuracy and precision.

Mistake 1

When you are learning the placement of a step, try not to get into the habit of looking down.

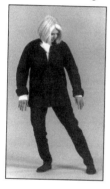

Mistake 2

Don't raise your shoulders as you raise your arms.

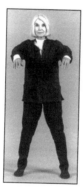

Mistake 3

If you do not release the toes (unhinge the gate) when you make the turn into the 70/30 Posture, you end up in a twisted, uncomfortable position—with your foot at a 90- instead of a 45-degree angle.

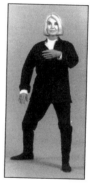

Mistake 4

As you shift all of your weight into the back leg, do not lean backward. Carry the entire upper body back as a single unit.

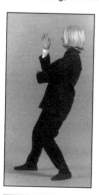

Mistake 5

Never lead with your hipbone. Move all the building blocks at once. If any part of your body protrudes from the rest, relax and realign.

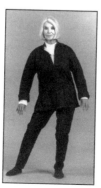

Mistake 6

As you step forward (with either foot), the tendency is to draw the front foot in close to the heel of the back foot. Instead, move the foot in an absolutely straight line so that the feet will be shoulder distance apart once you've made your turn and arrive in the 70/30 Posture.

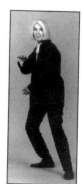

Mistake 7
Don't let your head anticipate where you are going and get ahead of the step. Nose over navel is the rule.

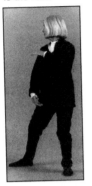

Mistake 8
Be careful not to lead with your chest, which will throw you off balance.

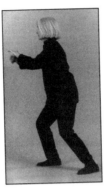

Mistake 9
Do not push forward by leading with your knee. The knee should not go beyond the toes.

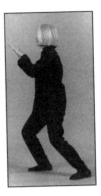

Mistake 10
Be sure to keep both knees equally bent. Never lock the knee joints.

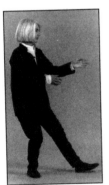

Mistake 11
Never break at the wrist. The shape from the fingers to the elbow always remains as one unbroken line.

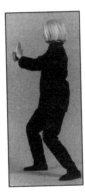

Mistake 12
When you are facing a corner and stepping out with either foot, be sure not to step too far forward or you will lose your balance and will need to throw weight into the leg before you have shifted 70 percent.

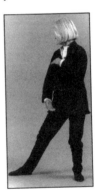

A FINAL WORD

Now that you've become familiar with the vocabulary of T'ai Chi Ch'uan and how the movements link one to the other, here are some additional ideas to explore that will deepen your comprehension of T'ai Chi.

Why not try the following:

1. Do the form once in a while with a book balanced on your head. This will tell you if you are truly aligned.

2. Practice any sections of the form you wish without using your arms and hands at all. Just move the lower part of your body. (You will see that all arm movements are initiated by the pelvis.)

3. Try coordinating your breath with the movements, inhaling as your arms move out and exhaling as your arms return and you root down into your legs.

4. Sometimes follow the flow of gentle, classical music as you perform the steps. This will soften the edges of your form.

5. Take one principle at a time—say, dropping your tailbone—and go through the form just making sure your sacrum is plumb-line straight to the ground.

6. During practice, but not while you are running through the entire twenty steps, hold a position and check the pertinent principles: Is your head straight? Is your chest deflated and directly over your pelvis? Is your tailbone dropped?

7. Watch your inner thoughts as you perform the steps. Is your mind wandering? With ease, bring your awareness back to the subtlety and intricacy of the movement at hand. (You will develop your powers of concentration as you practice.)

8. Stand with your back to a wall. Bend your legs at the groin almost to a right angle. Press each vertebra to the wall, starting from the coccyx and going up the spine to the back of the head. This will strengthen the small of your back and eliminate arching.

9. Stand next to a table with your body in correct alignment and hold on lightly with one hand. Then lift one foot off the ground and maintain that position as long as it is bearable (say, one to three minutes). Then change feet and balance on the other leg. Eventually do the exercise without holding onto a support.

10. Sit down quietly. Close your eyes. Wait. You will begin to feel a tingling (for some people a sensation of heat) perhaps first in your hands and arms but eventually in any part of your body where you place your thought. You are now in touch with the *ch'i* within you. As you experience more and more the *ch'i* circulating throughout your body, you will learn to direct the *ch'i* with your mind to sink down to the *tan-tien*. Mysterious as it sounds, *ch'i* power will accumulate there, and in time you will be able to move the *ch'i* to all parts of your body at will. You will then have entered a further dimension of health and strength.

Do not hurry your practice of T'ai Chi. There is a story told by the ancient Chinese sage Mencius to his students. Mencius said, "Let the mind not forget its objective, but let there be no artificial effort to help it grow. Do not be like the man of Sung. There was a man of Sung who was sorry that his corn was not growing, and so he pulled at the stalks. Having been tired out, he went home and said to his people, 'I am all tired. I have helped the corn to grow.' When his son ran to look at it, the corn had already withered."[3]

You cannot force the results of the T'ai Chi form. Your body has to go through the process of softening and becoming pliable. This takes time. With suppleness, you gain strength. With strength, you achieve the fluid balance needed to execute the movements. All of this takes more time. But the process *is* T'ai Chi. It is a never-ending process. And from the first day of practice, you will see and feel great changes in your physical well-being.

As you grasp the principles, apply them to your life outside of your daily practice. When you walk, stand, sit, catch a train, talk on the telephone, let this new way of being be felt in your entire body in all of your activities. This in turn will benefit your development in the form itself. Don't get frustrated by any initial awkwardness or a feeling that you are not progressing fast enough. Trust the Masters—each day you will be deepening the form. Even as a beginner, you will sense T'ai Chi reaching out, touching and informing all aspects of your life.

Be patient, have perseverance, and enjoy this incredible gift from the other side of the world.

3. Wing-Tsit Chan, *A Source Book in Chinese Philosophy* (Princeton University Press, 1963), p. 63.

T'ai Chi Short Form:
First Twenty Postures in
Continuous Sequence

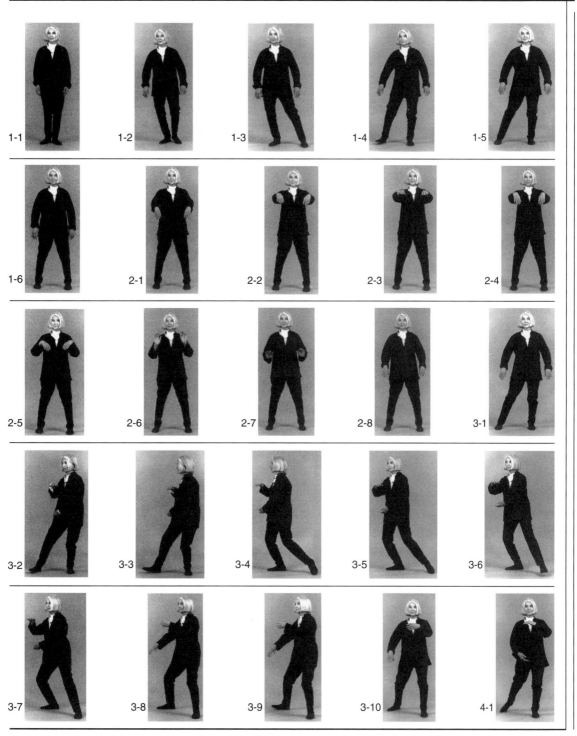

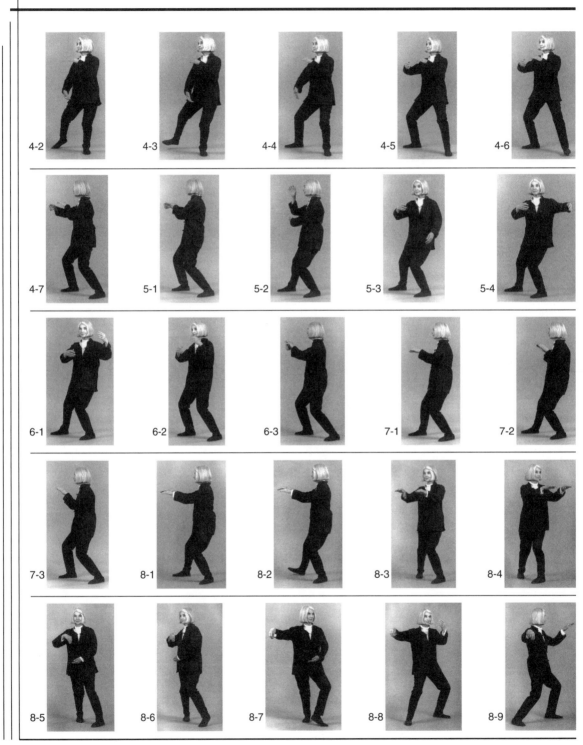

4-2 4-3 4-4 4-5 4-6

4-7 5-1 5-2 5-3 5-4

6-1 6-2 6-3 7-1 7-2

7-3 8-1 8-2 8-3 8-4

8-5 8-6 8-7 8-8 8-9

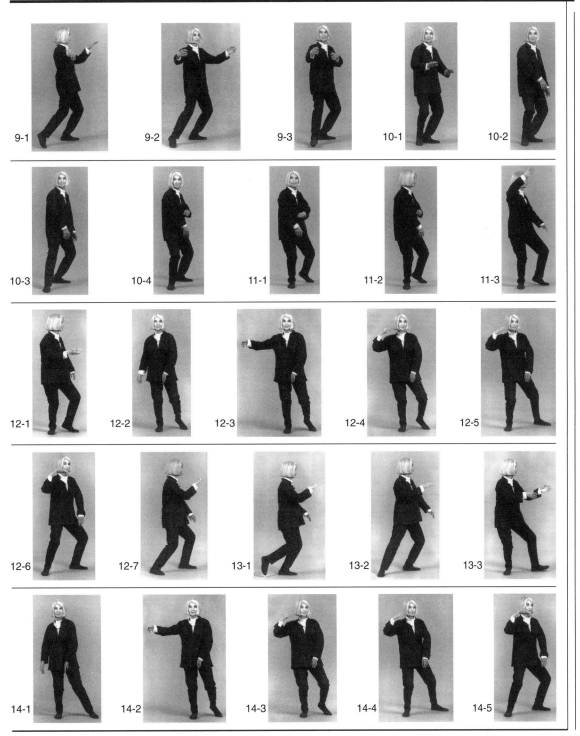

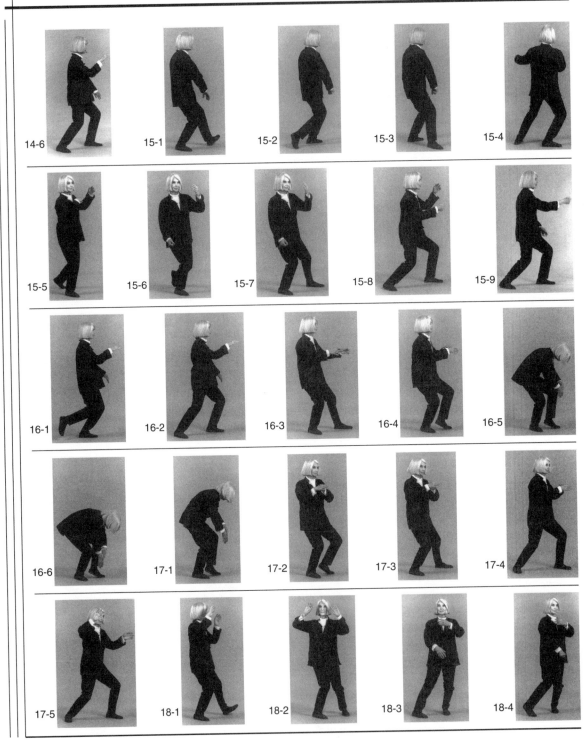

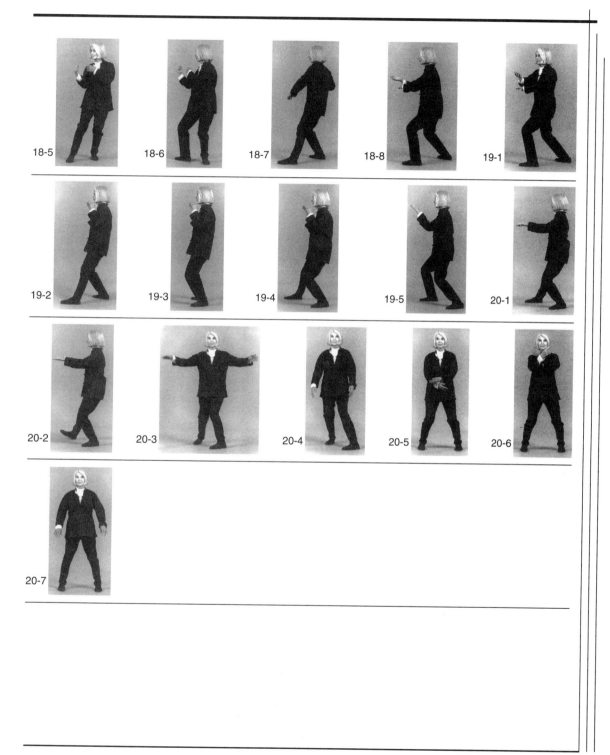

18-5   18-6   18-7   18-8   19-1

19-2   19-3   19-4   19-5   20-1

20-2   20-3   20-4   20-5   20-6

20-7

BIBLIOGRAPHY

Chen, William C. C. *Body Mechanics of Tai Chi Chuan*. William C. C. Chen, 1973.

Cheng Man-ch'ing and Robert W. Smith. *T'ai Chi*. Charles E. Tuttle Co., 1967.

Da Liu. *T'ai Chi Ch'uan & Meditation*. Schocken Books, 1986.

Delza, Sophia. *T'ai-Chi Ch'uan* (Wu style). State University of New York Press, 1985.

Galante, Lawrence. *Tai Chi*. Samuel Weiser, 1981.

Huang, Wen-Shan. *Fundamentals of T'ai Chi Ch'uan*. South Sky Book Co., 1973.

Kauz, Herman. *Tai Chi Handbook*. Doubleday, 1974.

Klein, Bob. *Movements of Magic*. Newcastle Publishing Co., 1984.

Kostias, John. *The Essential Movements of T'ai Chi*. Paradigm Publications, 1989.

Lao-tzu. *Tao Teh Ching*. Translated by Gia-Fu and Jane English. Alfred A. Knopf, 1974.

LaTourette, Kenneth Scott. *The Chinese—Their History and Culture*. Macmillan, 1962.

Lee Ying-arng. *Lee's Modified T'ai Chi for Health*. McLisa Enterprises, 1968.

Liao, Waysun. *T'ai Chi Classics*. Shambhala Publications, 1990.

Moyers, Bill. *Healing and the Mind*. Doubleday, 1993.

Sohn, Robert C. *Tao and T'ai Chi Kung*. Destiny Books, 1989.

Waley, Arthur. *The Way and Its Power*. Grove Press, 1958.

Wing-Tsit Chan. *A Source Book in Chinese Philosophy*. Princeton University Press, 1963.

Yang Jwing-Ming. *Tai Chi Chi Kung*. Yang's Martial Arts Association, 1990.

Yang Ming-Shi. *Tai Chi Chuan for Health and Beauty*. Bunka Publishing Bureau, 1976.

On videocassette: *Claire Hooton, T'ai Chi for Health & Fitness,* available in beginner and intermediate levels. Both programs offer easy-to-follow instruction on the postures embodied in the Yang-style Short Form.

Available in all major video stores, or, to order, call 1-800-272-4214 between 8:30 and 4:45 EST, or write to

Parade Video, 88 St. Francis St., Newark, NJ 07105.